The Renfrew Unified Treatment for Eating Disorders and Comorbidity

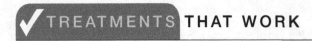 TREATMENTS THAT WORK

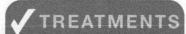 **TREATMENTS** THAT WORK

The Renfrew Unified Treatment for Eating Disorders and Comorbidity

An Adaptation of the Unified Protocol

WORKBOOK

HEATHER THOMPSON-BRENNER
MELANIE SMITH
GAYLE BROOKS
DEE ROSS FRANKLIN
HALLIE ESPEL-HUYNH
JAMES F. BOSWELL

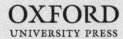
OXFORD
UNIVERSITY PRESS

OXFORD
UNIVERSITY PRESS

Oxford University Press is a department of the University of Oxford. It furthers the University's objective of excellence in research, scholarship, and education by publishing worldwide. Oxford is a registered trade mark of Oxford University Press in the UK and certain other countries.

Published in the United States of America by Oxford University Press
198 Madison Avenue, New York, NY 10016, United States of America.

Library of Congress Cataloging-in-Publication Data
Names: Thompson-Brenner, Heather, editor.
Title: The Renfrew unified treatment for eating disorders and comorbidity : an adaptation of the unified protocol, workbook / [edited by] Heather Thompson-Brenner,
Melanie Smith, Gayle Brooks, Dee Ross Franklin, Hallie Espel-Huynh, James F. Boswell.
Description: New York, NY : Oxford University Press, 2021. |
Series: Treatments that work series | Includes bibliographical references and index.
Identifiers: LCCN 2020056413 (print) | LCCN 2020056414 (ebook) |
ISBN 9780190947002 (paperback) | ISBN 9780190947026 (epub) | ISBN 9780190947033
Subjects: LCSH: Eating disorders—Treatment. | Comorbidity.
Classification: LCC RC552.E18 R522 2021 (print) |
LCC RC552.E18 (ebook) | DDC 616.85/26—dc23
LC record available at https://lccn.loc.gov/2020056413
LC ebook record available at https://lccn.loc.gov/2020056414

DOI: 10.1093/med-psych/9780190947002.001.0001

One of the most difficult problems confronting patients with various disorders and diseases is finding the best help available. Everyone is aware of friends or family who have sought treatment from a seemingly reputable practitioner only to find out later from another doctor that the original diagnosis was wrong or the treatments recommended were inappropriate or perhaps even harmful. Most patients, or family members, address this problem by reading everything they can about their symptoms, seeking out information on the internet, or actively "asking around" to tap knowledge from friends and acquaintances. Governments and healthcare policymakers are also aware that people in need don't always get the best treatments—something they refer to as "variability in healthcare practices."

Healthcare systems around the world are now attempting to correct this variability by introducing "evidence-based practice." This simply means that it is in everyone's interest that patients get the most up-to-date and effective care for a particular problem. Healthcare policymakers have also recognized that it is very useful to give consumers of healthcare as much information as possible, so that they can make intelligent decisions in a collaborative effort to improve physical health and mental health. This series, *Treatments ThatWork*™, is designed to accomplish just that. Only the latest and most effective interventions for particular problems are described, written in user-friendly language. To be included in this series, each treatment program must pass the highest standards of evidence available, as determined by a scientific advisory board. Thus, when individuals suffering from these problems or their family members seek out an expert clinician who is familiar with these interventions and decides that they are appropriate, they will have confidence that they are receiving the best care available. Of course, only your healthcare professional can decide on the right mix of treatments for you.

This workbook is designed for your use as you work with a qualified mental health professional to address your eating disorder and other co-occurring emotional issues, such as anxiety and depression. It presents a step-by-step approach for addressing your individual eating issues as well as your particular mood or anxiety problems, using an integrated set of flexible tools. These tools are based on the principles of cognitive-behavioral therapy as well as other therapeutic interventions that have demonstrated effectiveness in research studies for both eating disorders and other emotional disorders. Each chapter builds on skills explained and learned in previous chapters, so we suggest that you progress through them in sequence. We suggest, as much as possible, that you read the relevant chapter and attempt to complete the exercises in that chapter before you meet with your therapist. Over the course of the program you will learn to understand the relationship between your eating behaviors and emotions, and work through the problems you experience by identifying and challenging relevant thoughts. Through exposure exercises designed to help you with challenging situations, the program should help you overcome these problems in a safe, structured way. If you are motivated, and if you are able to put in the time and effort, you are likely to find this program will help improve your quality of life.

David H. Barlow, Editor-in-Chief
Treatments ThatWork™
Boston, MA

Contents

Acknowledgments

We would like to express our deep gratitude to individuals and groups who supported the development and study of this treatment program. First, we want to acknowledge that this treatment is itself an adaptation of another treatment, which in turn is comprised of core elements of psychotherapy that have worked across different populations for a wide range of emotional issues. There are many unique and creative aspects to every treatment manual, but the entire field of psychotherapy research has contributed to identifying and refining the treatment strategies that are presented here. More specifically, however, we would like to express our appreciation for the following individuals who were essential to the process of adapting, implementing, refining, and studying this protocol. At the Renfrew Center, we want to mention Sam Menaged, Susan Ice, Michael Lowe, Amy Banks, Taylor Gardner, Shelby Ortiz, Alex Goncalves, Heather Maio, Adrienne Ressler, Christina Felonis, and Rachel Dore. Many other important people have contributed to the work at the Renfrew Center and at Boston University, and were essential to the success of the program and the eventual publication of this manual. We would all like to acknowledge our families, as well, who have supported us through everything.

Preparing for Treatment

CHAPTER 1

Eating Disorders and Emotional Disorders

- Describe the types of problems this program was designed to address.
- Help you determine whether your difficulties fit with this program.
- Understand how eating disorders and other emotional disorders occur together.

Eating disorders and emotions

This treatment is designed to address any type of eating disorder along with the other emotional problems that people with eating disorders also commonly experience. Eating disorders are related to emotional functioning in many important ways. First, negative emotions—and the desire to avoid or control negative emotions—have been shown repeatedly to be related to the development of eating disorders as well as to most other emotional disorders. Depression and anxiety are known risk factors for the development of an eating disorder. Research also shows that emotional events—such as feeling sadness, feeling anxiety, or feeling stress—are often the immediate triggers for eating disorder symptoms. Furthermore, having an eating disorder is a difficult emotional experience, and many people develop depression and anxiety in reaction to their eating disorder symptoms. So, emotions create the context in which eating disorders develop, emotions are a part of what drives eating disorder symptoms on a daily level, and emotional experiences become worse as a result of having an eating disorder.

This workbook was developed to help people who have eating disorders and who are also struggling with intense and difficult emotions like anxiety, sadness, anger, and guilt. When people have both an eating disorder and another disorder, like anxiety or depression, we call this "co-occurring disorders," or more than one disorder going on at the same time. For the purposes of this treatment, we consider eating disorders to be a particular type of emotional disorder, with some symptoms focused in the areas of eating and body image. Everyone has difficult emotions that are intense at times. We call patterns of negative emotions a "disorder," however, when the emotions are so intense and difficult that they get in the way of living life. For example, *shame* and *anxiety* about eating can prevent people from spending time with friends or developing new relationships. *Sadness* can make it hard to go to school or work, or even get out of bed. You may have picked up this book because eating symptoms and emotions are interfering in your own life in ways that matter to you. Although emotions affect our lives in different ways, there are three features that often occur in all emotional disorders:

1. **Frequent, strong emotions**: People who end up with the symptoms of emotional disorders tend to feel strong emotions quite often. This is often a biological tendency to be emotionally sensitive—some people may simply be hardwired to experience their emotions more intensely in response to situations in their lives. It is important to point out, though, that feeling emotions strongly does not necessarily mean that the person will find them distressing or interfering. It is how we respond to our emotions that really matters.

2. **Negative reactions to emotions**: People with emotional disorders also tend to view their emotions negatively. They can be hard on themselves for having certain reactions, thinking "I shouldn't be feeling this way" or "Getting upset about this is a sign of weakness." They also may link strong emotions to bad outcomes and conclude things like, "Everyone will judge me for being anxious," "If I get angry, I'll do something that I regret," or "If I let myself feel sad, I'll fall into a hole that I won't be able to get out of." Sometimes one part of an emotional experience is particularly distressing. For example, some people may find the physical sensations associated with emotions—like a racing heart, sweating, and nausea or stomach pain—very difficult to bear. Sometimes people even have negative reactions to positive emotions. For example, they might think, "If I let myself feel hopeful or excited, I'll be even more disappointed if it doesn't work out."

3. **Avoidance of emotions**: Since people with emotional disorders view their emotions negatively, it makes sense that they would try to avoid them. The problem with avoidance is that it actually doesn't work well over the long term. Actively trying to push away emotions may make you feel better in the short term, but it generally leads to more frequent, intense emotions in the long term. It is like being stuck in quicksand—the more you struggle, the more you sink. Additionally, by avoiding activities or situations because they might bring up intense emotions, life can become limited. You may find it difficult to get the most out of important day-to-day activities like going to work, spending time with friends, or just doing something fun. Missing out on life also adds to people's negative emotions. People with eating disorders have often gone through a time of having intense negative emotions—such as in adolescence, around school, or after the breakup of a relationship—and find that controlling their eating or losing weight helps them avoid those emotions and even feel a little better for a while. However, the negative emotions usually return, new ones may develop, and physical and medical symptoms may arise around eating symptoms.

The goal of this workbook is to change the way you respond to your emotions when they occur. Specifically, you will be asked to approach your emotions in a more accepting manner instead of viewing them as something to avoid. This may seem like the opposite of what you were expecting; perhaps you are hoping to get rid of your overwhelming emotions. However, as you progress through this workbook, you will learn more about how emotions, even negative ones, are important, and that pushing them away actually backfires. Leaning in toward your emotions and responding more effectively to them may be difficult at first, but it will gradually make your emotions more manageable.

To begin to see if this program is right for you, take a look at these examples of people we have treated in our programs.

Samantha

Samantha is a 21-year-old college student who came to our clinic for help with co-occurring problems with eating and emotions. Samantha first noticed she had problems with her emotions in high school. She was a high-achieving student-athlete, but she became anxious and perfectionistic, and went through a time when she had difficulty sleeping and finishing her projects on time because she was so nervous that she would make a mistake. Samantha was admitted to a good college, but in her first semester, she noticed that her difficulty worrying about her coursework and homework assignments had returned even stronger, and she became anxious about what her professors and other students were thinking about her. She had decided to stop playing sports so she could focus on academics, and then she found she was waking up early to work out, skipping meals, and adding another workout at night in hopes that the exercise would make her feel less anxious and better about herself in general. Samantha became very tired, less interested in socializing than usual, and sad. She noticed it became harder to concentrate—she kept thinking about her worries, and she experienced intrusive thoughts about food and exercise. She felt hopeless about achieving what she wanted in school and started worrying that her professors would think she should never have been admitted to her program. When Samantha went home for the holidays, her parents were startled at her appearance and very concerned. Her doctor told her she had lost a large amount of weight, her blood pressure was low, and she was suffering from malnutrition.

Andrew

Andrew is an 18-year-old high school senior. When Andrew was in middle school, his classmates made fun of him for being "fat." He spent a lot of time looking at himself in the mirror early in high school, examining the acne that he hated on his face. He avoided social gatherings and dating, worrying that others would find him ugly and disgusting. In his junior year, he told his best friend that he had fallen in love. Unfortunately, however, that person did not return his romantic affection. Andrew couldn't shake the sadness and feelings of shame and started to stay home from school, saying that he was "sick." Over the course of a few months, without thinking about it, he lost some weight. When his family pushed him to return to school, some of his friends told him he looked good. He decided to avoid eating for a while, following a "fasting" diet he read about online. Andrew lost more weight and started exercising, and soon had lost a substantial amount of weight. He started to find, however, that after a day of fasting, he would lose control of his eating at night, and he eventually begin binge eating large amounts of food and then vomiting to make himself feel better. During the days after a binge episode, Andrew would feel intense shame and embarrassment, believing that others could see a change in his appearance, would know that he had been binge eating, and would think he was fat. He began to spend more time checking in the mirror to see whether his waist and face looked "right," sometimes hours at a time.

As his binge eating and purging increased in frequency, his depression became more intense.

Rani

Rani is a 41-year-old, married mother of two children who works in the medical industry. Rani was the youngest child in a large family, and one of her older siblings had a severe medical illness. Rani felt that her role in the family was to help her mother and her sister to function, or else things might fall apart. Rani was a nervous child and found herself obsessing about particular worries such as choking, vomiting, or getting sick. Her years as a graduate student and young wife were happy and busy. After the birth of her second child, however, she found that her old worries became more severe. She washed her hands frequently, avoided touching her hands to her mouth, and eventually began avoiding all foods that she felt could have germs on them. She often noticed that she had stomach pains and diarrhea, and though her primary care doctor couldn't find a medical problem, Rani thought she might have food intolerances or irritable bowel syndrome. Rani started making her plans around being near a bathroom at all times and eliminated foods with gluten and dairy from her diet. When she returned to work after an extended maternity leave, it became so difficult to manage her routine of washing her hands, and washing and preparing her food, that she decided it was easier to stop eating at all during the day. At work, she found herself on the verge of a panic attack several times a week—her anxiety symptoms included tightness in her throat and nausea, and these feelings were scarily like choking or being ill. When she stopped having her period, she again worried this might be a symptom of a severe illness, but her friends suggested it could be the beginning of menopause. When she consulted a gynecologist, she was surprised to learn that anxiety and food restriction, such as she had been experiencing, was actually an eating disorder and could cause amenorrhea (loss of normal menstrual cycle).

Deneice

Deneice is a 32-year-old emergency dispatcher. Her parents struggled with substance abuse, and her father died from a heart attack when she was a girl. Her mother then had difficulty managing the stresses of single parenthood, along with her personal problems, and Deneice often found herself in scary situations on her own. Two times in high school she was sexually assaulted after she had too much to drink. As an adult, she worked very hard to get her life together and was proud of her strong academic record and excellent job performance. After long hours of exhausting and stressful work, Deneice liked to watch television and eat comforting food, often past the point of feeling full. She figured that "emotional eating" was less problematic than the substance abuse her parents had suffered from, though she worried about her weight, particularly given her family history of cardiovascular disease. One night her apartment was broken into, and she found herself face to face with an intruder. She froze, and the man ran away without harming her further. After the break-in, however, Deneice started to have terrifying dreams and trouble sleeping. She worried that another intruder would break in and that she would not be able to defend herself. She moved to a new apartment with a high-tech security system and made sure she had several different phones charged and ready in case she faced a similar situation. As her anxiety increased, she began to feel claustrophobic and stopped going to movies, riding on the subway, or being in crowded situations where she might have the terrible feelings she had experienced during the break-in. When she had to be in crowds or otherwise uncomfortable situations, she would repeatedly check the exits and would keep her phone in her hand. Driving became stressful, and it was difficult to get to work. Her job dealing with other people's emergencies became too stressful, and after speaking with human resources, she began working on the application for a medical leave of absence; she then found that the prospect of being out of work and isolated in her apartment was even more frightening than trying to manage her daily routine. As her exhaustion increased, alone in her apartment at night, Deneice found her eating became more and more out of control. She ate to the point of feeling sick, and she felt guilty and ashamed during the day. She tried to make a plan to take care of herself, but at night she would repeatedly find herself ordering food or driving to the grocery store, sometimes barely aware that she was doing it.

You may notice that each person just described is experiencing different symptoms. In each of these cases, however, strong emotions and eating problems are getting in the way of their ability to live the life they want. Their negative reactions to their emotions are driving them to do things they don't want to do. And as we will discuss throughout this program, things that might make them feel better for a short time—such as skipping social gatherings, avoiding crowds, restricting food, or binge eating—actually lead to more problems in the long term. All of these problems may feel like terrible traps. However, this treatment program includes many tools to help change these patterns.

Many programs to treat eating disorders, or other emotional disorders, start with working on just one disorder, with the hope that any other problems a person has will get better when one big part of the problem is removed. As we said earlier, it is very common that people with eating disorders also have at least one other serious emotional disorder, such as anxiety or depression. Sometimes this one-issue-at-a-time approach works. However, eating disorders and co-occurring emotional disorders have very important patterns in common, and we have found that it can be more powerful to treat the issues in combination, understanding them together, and dealing with everything at the same time, using a unified approach.

This treatment is designed to help people like Samantha, Andrew, Rani, and Deneice. By focusing on negative, avoidant reactions to strong emotions, we can help people with a variety of different problems. There are a variety of mental health conditions that can be considered emotional disorders and would be a good fit for this treatment. As a reminder, emotional disorders occur when the way a person responds to strong emotions is taking over his or her life. Examples of emotional disorders include eating disorders, anxiety disorders, posttraumatic stress disorder, and obsessive-compulsive disorder. Depression is another common emotional disorder. Table 1.1 lists many diagnoses and problems that are characterized by difficulties responding to strong emotions.

You may have visited a mental health professional and received one of more of these diagnoses. In fact, it is actually quite common for people to have more than one disorder at the same time. This is because the same process—negative reactions to strong emotions—is a part of all emotional disorders and related problems, such as self-injury and substance abuse. This is an important reason why we developed the treatment program here. By focusing on negative, avoidant reactions to emotions, we can help you address all the symptoms you are experiencing, regardless of the disorder.

Even if you have not received one of these diagnoses, this program might still be a good fit for you. If your emotions (or the strategies you use to manage them) are interfering with living the life you want to lead, you will probably benefit from the skills taught in this workbook. For some people, strong emotions affect nearly every aspect of their lives, while for others, difficulties with emotions only occur in one or two areas.

Table 1.1 Eating Disorders and Emotional Disorders

Eating disorder diagnoses

Anorexia Nervosa (AN)	People with AN deliberately restrict their food intake and have a low body weight for their height. People with AN often have a strong fear of gaining weight. Their fear of gaining weight drives them to restrict their overall food intake, to avoid particular foods that inspire that fear, and to over-exercise or take other measures to avoid weight gain. The fear of gaining weight can make it difficult for people with AN to fully appreciate the serious medical consequences of malnutrition or to address these consequences. The consequences of malnutrition can also include difficulty concentrating, depression, sleeplessness, and anxiety. Malnutrition can also cause binge eating, which in turn can cause extreme fear of weight gain.
Bulimia Nervosa (BN)	People with BN experience episodes where they lose control of their eating, which causes intense feelings of shame and guilt, and they then engage in "compensatory" behaviors to address the effects of binge eating, such as purging by vomiting, taking laxatives or diet pills, and obsessive exercise to reduce those emotions. Individuals with BN also often restrict their food intake or avoid certain foods. Individuals with BN report that they have intense negative feelings associated with their dissatisfaction with their bodies, as well as fear of gaining weight. Dieting and engaging in compensatory behaviors can temporarily reduce negative emotions; however, they can be dangerous, and they also make it more likely that the binge eating will occur more frequently and more intensely.
Binge Eating Disorder (BED)	People with BED experience episodes where they lose control of their eating, followed by intense feelings of shame and guilt. Some people with BED are very dissatisfied with their body shape or weight. People with BED very commonly experience anxiety disorders and depression.
Avoidant-Restrictive Food Intake Disorder (ARFID)	People with ARFID restrict their food intake to the point of being underweight and risking medical consequences of malnutrition; however, they do not do so out of a fear of gaining weight or body dissatisfaction. There are several common emotional issues associated with ARFID, including extreme negative reactions to the taste or texture of certain foods, and certain phobias such as choking phobia or fear of vomiting, and other anxiety disorders. People with ARFID avoid eating because of the negative emotions they anticipate having in response to eating; however, as with AN, they can suffer medical consequences, depression, difficulty concentrating, and other problems as a result of malnutrition.

Emotional disorders that commonly co-occur with eating disorders

Panic Disorder (PD)	People with PD have panic attacks—sudden rushes of intense fear with uncomfortable physical sensations (for example, racing heart, sweating, dizziness, shortness of breath). People with PD find these experiences extremely distressing and attempt to avoid them at all costs. This avoidance may look like staying away from any place where a panic attack might happen, refraining from taking the bus or subway, and avoiding caffeinated drinks. Avoiding particular places outside the home, because they might lead to a panic attack, is called *agoraphobia*.

Table 1.1 Continued

Generalized Anxiety Disorder (GAD)	People with GAD engage in a great deal of worry about all sorts of topics—for example, being on time, finances, the health of themselves or loved ones, social issues, or work/school. Often this worry is future-oriented and is out of proportion to the severity of the topic. Once they get started worrying, they find it very difficult to stop. People with GAD will often do things to make themselves feel better, like calling to check in on loved ones, checking bank balances, over-preparing or procrastinating, and searching for information on the internet. Unfortunately, these behaviors make people with GAD feel better for only a short time and often backfire.
Social Anxiety Disorder (SAD)	People with SAD experience anxiety in situations where they might be observed or evaluated by others. In order to avoid these feelings, they might refrain from entering situations where other people are present (for example, going to parties, the lunchroom, or the mall) or situations where they might have to speak up (for example, taking classes with a public speaking component). They may also try to reduce their anxiety by avoiding eye contact, avoiding disagreeing with other people, or only talking about topics they know a lot about. These behaviors may make people with SAD feel better in the moment, but they lend support to the belief that others may be judging them.
Obsessive-Compulsive Disorder (OCD)	OCD is characterized by intrusive thoughts (obsessions) that often seem nonsensical (for example, "I'll get HIV from touching this door knob") but cause a great deal of distress. Often people with OCD engage in behaviors to manage the thoughts (compulsions). These behaviors and rituals can be time-consuming and disruptive (for example, repeated handwashing), but people with OCD keep doing them because they reduce the distress caused by the obsessions, at least for a short while. Unfortunately, reacting to these thoughts as if they could be true, by engaging in compulsions, makes it more likely that these thoughts will return in the future.
Posttraumatic Stress disorder (PTSD)	Some people who have experienced a traumatic event (assault, combat, abuse) develop PTSD. This disorder is characterized by intrusive memories of the event that the individual finds quite distressing. As a result, people with PTSD avoid triggers (people, situations, activities that remind them of the trauma). They may also engage in behaviors that make them feel safe in general (for example, having an exit strategy, or always facing the door). Unfortunately, acting as though they are still in danger can reinforce and increase their distress.
Major Depressive Disorder (MDD)	People with MDD report feelings of sadness and hopelessness. They often have little energy or motivation to do the things they used to find fun. They may lack appetite or may experience unusually strong urges to eat, and they often feel fatigued and have trouble with too much or too little sleep. Although getting active has been shown to help people with depression, it is extremely difficult for people with depression to "get over the hump." As a result, they tend to withdraw by canceling plans and avoiding important activities. Although this avoidance brings some relief in the short term, it has been shown to increase symptoms of depression.

(continued)

11

Table 1.1 Continued

Body Dysmorphic Disorder (BDD)	People with BDD believe that there is something terribly wrong with their appearance, though other people do not perceive the same flaws. People with BDD spend a lot of time checking on their appearance and trying to alter their appearance in order to change or disguise their perceived flaws. They may also go to great lengths to avoid seeing themselves or having other people see their bodies. Though checking and avoidance may temporarily provide reassurance or relief, the amount of time spent engaging in these behaviors can actually strengthen the belief or perception that something is terribly wrong.
Borderline Personality Disorder (BPD)	People with BPD report feeling all of their emotions really strongly—in fact, they are often described as moody because their feelings can change quite quickly. To manage their negative emotions, people with BPD engage in a wide range of behaviors that make them feel better in the moment but lead to even more problems in the longer term. These behaviors include picking fights with people, seeking excessive reassurance in relationships, binge eating, drug use, and self-injury.
Substance Use Disorders (SUDs)	Substance use disorders are complicated behavioral, impulse-control, and genetic disorders, and they also have a component that is related to emotional avoidance. Individuals with SUDs sometimes report that they use substances to numb or avoid negative feelings. Even when the disorder does not start that way, people with substance problems accumulate negative feelings associated with their substance use and the problems that it causes, and then report that they use substances to avoid these feelings of self-judgment and guilt over time. Recovery from SUDs can involve identifying negative emotions and learning to tolerate them instead of avoiding them through substance abuse.
Self-Destructive Behaviors	While self-destructive behaviors do not necessarily constitute a mental health diagnosis, they are often used to provide temporary relief from negative emotions. These behaviors can include things like self-injury (for example, cutting or burning oneself on purpose), excessive drinking or substance use, lashing out or snapping at others, and other reckless behaviors. These behaviors may take someone's mind off of their emotions in the short term but can lead to negative consequences, and even more negative emotions, in the longer term.

How was this treatment program tested?

This program has been tested in many research studies. The original program, called the "Unified Protocol," was created by combining different elements of treatment to address emotional problems in hundreds of studies. The combined treatment, which uses these combined approaches to address emotional avoidance and emotional acceptance, was then tested in several large studies for people with depression and anxiety disorders. The research studies showed that the treatment program was very effective for a range of different emotional disorders and just as effective for their primary diagnosis as other state-of-the-art single-disorder treatments. The program was then adapted by clinicians and researchers at The Renfrew Center. It was adapted to be used with clients with all the eating disorder diagnoses, adjusted to be easy to use in groups as well as in individual treatment, and modified to be used across multiple levels of care, including residential treatment, day hospital, and outpatient treatment. As it was adapted for use with clients with eating disorders in The Renfrew Center, it was also adapted to be usable by clients who have very severe problems, and an additional focus on the relationship between the therapist and the client, and between clients in group treatment, was also added. This adapted treatment for eating disorders and co-occurring emotional disorders, published in this workbook, is called the "Unified Treatment" (UT). Several large research studies conducted by researchers working with The Renfrew Center have shown that the UT was more effective than the treatment that was being used in the period before the UT was developed and implemented in two residential programs. Follow-up research showed that the UT did work by the methods that it was intended to—that people who received the UT became more emotionally accepting and less avoidant of emotions, and that these changes were related to the changes that were observed in eating disorder symptoms. Other follow-up research shows that these improvements in the effectiveness of treatment are still seen in clients at The Renfrew Center in the several years that have passed, and in the hundreds of clients who have been treated, since the time the UT was developed and began to be used.

References

Research on the Unified Treatment

Thompson-Brenner, H., Boswell, J. F., Espel-Huynh, H., Brooks, G. E., & Lowe, M. R. (2019). Implementation of transdiagnostic treatment for emotional disorders in residential eating disorder programs: A preliminary pre-post evaluation. *Psychotherapy Research*, *29*(8), 1045–1061.

Thompson-Brenner, H., Brooks, G. E., Boswell, J. F., Espel-Huynh, H. M., Dore, R., Franklin, D. R., Gonçalves, A., Smith, M., Ortiz, S., Ice, S., Barlow, D. H., & Lowe, M. R. (2018). Evidence-based implementation practices applied to the intensive treatment of eating disorders: A research summary and examples from one case. *Clinical Psychology: Science and Practice*, *25*(1), e12221.

Thompson-Brenner, H., Singh, S., Gardner, T., Brooks, G. E., Smith, M.T., Lowe , M.R., Boswell, J.F. (2021). The renfrew unified treatment for eating disorders and comorbidity: Long-term effects of an evidence-based practice implementation in residential treatment. *Frontiers in Psychiatry*, *12*, 226.

Research on the Unified Protocol

Barlow, D. H., Farchione, T. J., Bullis, J. R., Gallagher, M. W., Murray-Latin, H., Sauer-Zavala, S., Bentley, K. H., Thompson-Hollands, J., Conklin, L. R., Boswell, J. F., Ametaj, A., Carl, J. R., Boettcher, H. T., & Cassiello-Robbins, C. F. (2017). The Unified Protocol for Transdiagnostic Treatment of Emotional Disorders compared with diagnosis-specific protocols for anxiety disorders: A randomized clinical trial. *JAMA Psychiatry, 74*(9), 875–884.

Barlow, D. H., Farchione, T. J., Fairholme, C. P., Ellard, K. K., Boisseau, C. L., & Allen, L. B. (2011). *Unified Protocol for Transdiagnostic Treatment of Emotional Disorders: Therapist guide.* Oxford University Press.

Farchione, T. J., Fairholme, C. P., Ellard, K. K., Boisseau, C. L., Thompson-Hollands, J., Carl, J. R., Gallagher, M. W., & Barlow, D. H. (2012). Unified Protocol for Transdiagnostic Treatment of Emotional Disorders: A randomized controlled trial. *Behavior Therapy, 43*(3), 666–678.

CHAPTER 2 About This Treatment

GOALS

- Provide an overview of the skills you will learn in this treatment.
- Highlight the importance of practicing these skills.
- Describe how this treatment can be used in combination with other treatments like medication, nutrition counseling, and other forms of therapy.
- Determine if now is the right time to begin this program.

In the previous chapter, we discussed some of the problems that this treatment can address. Now let's explore whether this treatment program is right for you.

Outline of the treatment

Each chapter of this workbook will teach you new skills to manage your emotions. As a reminder, the overall goal of this treatment is for you to become more accepting of your emotions in order to respond to them in more productive ways.

You can think of building a healthier relationship with your emotions as similar to building a new house, as illustrated in Figure 2.1.

You have to start by laying a solid foundation. There are three layers to this foundation that make up the initial, preparatory steps of treatment:

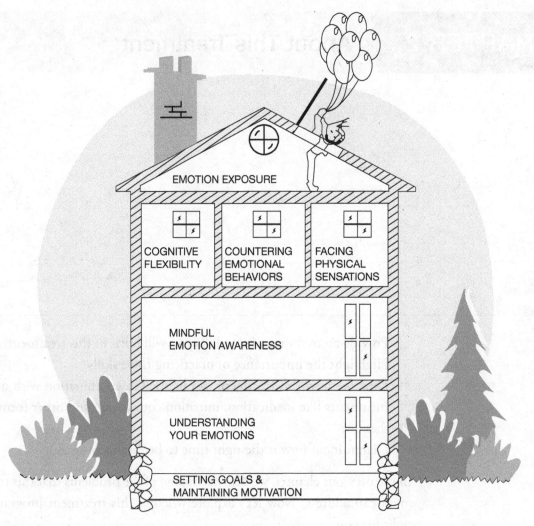

Figure 2.1:

Building a Healthy Relationship with Emotions: The Skills of the UT

- The first layer of this foundation is the skill of observing yourself objectively over time. In Chapter 3 you will learn about the power of self-monitoring to benefit your process of change.
- The second layer of this foundation, covered in Chapter 4, is identifying your personal reasons for making the changes outlined in this program in order to help you motivate yourself to put your best effort into developing these skills.
- In addition to being motivated and self-monitoring, many eating disorder research studies have suggested that early change in eating behavior is a very strong predictor of outcome. Therefore, Chapter 5 presents the goal of "regular eating" (three meals and three snacks

a day). It is very difficult to observe emotions and make changes in emotions without also eating somewhat regularly. You may already be eating regularly, and may also receive regular nutritional counseling, or even participate in structured meal programs, so this third goal may be less important for you to address as homework. However, it is an important part of the foundation for everyone with eating disorders.

After solidifying the necessary foundation for success, the ground floor of this program, which rests on the foundations, involves developing a greater understanding of your own emotional experiences:

- Given that accepting and approaching emotions may sound very different than what you expect, in Chapter 6 we discuss why we humans have emotions in the first place, and how they actually help us.
- In Chapter 7 we teach you to break down your emotions into more manageable parts. Specifically, we ask you to pay attention to your thoughts (what you tell yourself), physical sensations (what you feel in your body), and behaviors (what you do).
- Chapter 8 then teaches how to observe yourself objectively and understand how emotions can escalate and become overwhelming.

We will continue talking about these three parts of an emotion (thoughts, physical sensations, and behaviors), and how they interact and unfold over time, throughout this treatment.

After we have discussed why it makes sense to accept emotions as they come up, rather than avoid or escape from them, we will teach you a skill that will help you relate to your emotions in a more accepting way. The skill is called mindful emotion awareness and is covered in Chapter 9. You can think of this like going up to the second floor of the house to gain a different perspective on your emotional experiences. Specifically, we will ask you to look down on your thoughts, physical sensations, and behaviors in a nonjudgmental way. In other words, you will practice going easier on yourself for having emotional reactions—and just be aware of them, as they are—because beating yourself up only makes you feel worse! We will practice being nonjudgmentally aware of emotions through the exercise of mood induction (Chapter 10).

The next step will be to zero in on each of the three components of an emotion: thoughts, physical sensations, and behaviors. These three components each occupy a room on the third floor of our house, and behind each door is a new coping skill:

- You will learn how the way you think about situations in your life can really color how you feel about them. We will teach you a skill called cognitive flexibility (in Chapters 11 and 12) that will encourage you to question your first impressions so that you can think about things in a more balanced way.
- Next, we will focus on a skill called countering emotional behaviors (in Chapters 13 and 14). Here we ask you to begin to act in ways that approach emotions rather than pushing them away.
- Finally, in Chapter 15 you will learn a skill called understanding and confronting physical sensations. We will discuss the way that physical sensations contribute to how you experience emotions. We will also teach you exercises that will help you become more comfortable experiencing the physical sensations that go along with your emotions.

After you have learned skills to cope with strong emotions, it is important to put them into practice. The best way to do this is by facing situations or activities that bring up strong emotions. We call these practices emotion exposures and discuss these in Chapter 16. In addition to helping you practice your new skills, emotion exposures will allow you to learn important information about emotions themselves. By facing emotions, we learn that they are temporary and that we can actually tolerate them much better than we thought we could. Learning this firsthand (versus reading about it in a workbook) is the most powerful way to develop an accepting attitude toward emotions. This is the pinnacle of treatment and occupies the penthouse floor of our building.

We end with Chapter 17, "Continuing Progress into the Future," which is dedicated to making sure that you maintain the gains you made throughout your hard work with this treatment.

How should you use this workbook and treatment program?

This workbook and program are intended to be used in the context of therapy or counseling. There is also a complementary therapist manual with additional advice for professionals. The materials in this book may well be helpful to people who utilize them on their own, as self-help, but it has not yet been tested that way.

The treatment is designed to be flexible. In research studies and in a large number of treatment centers nationally, the treatment has been used in both individual and group therapy. This workbook is designed to be used in both types of therapy or counseling. In individual therapy, you can go at your own pace, spending enough time on each chapter to really become comfortable using the skills. In group therapy, the pace will be determined by the collective progress, your personal progress, and the assessment of the therapist. You can always continue to focus on a particular skill area in homework and revisit it in group discussion.

Each chapter has exercises that help you practice the skills in response to strong emotions in your life. There are exercises to complete in session—exercises that work in individual therapy or group therapy—or as homework. We recommend that you read the chapter and get started on the exercises prior to the session in which you will be working on the skill. However, your therapist can also review the psychoeducational material in session before leading the exercises.

Practice is extremely important. Reading the book and talking in therapy sessions are not enough—you have to make real changes in how you respond to your emotions in order to see improvements in how you feel. This involves doing homework between sessions, which may be challenging both in terms of the time it takes and the activities you are asked to do. Think of it like deciding to enter a marathon. You can't just sign up and expect to be able to run 26 miles. You have to exercise regularly to build up the strength to carry you through. This is why we discuss setting goals and maintaining motivation (Chapter 4) to make sure you are ready to fully commit to this program.

Can you do this treatment at the same time as doing other treatments?

This treatment is designed to be used in combination with nutrition counseling and psychiatry, if recommended by your therapist. In the major studies of this treatment, nutrition counseling and psychiatry were also received by clients. Crucially, however, the nutrition counseling and psychiatry sessions were designed to be compatible with this emotion-focused treatment that promotes emotional acceptance and works through reducing emotional and behavioral avoidance. Other forms of treatment and other approaches to counseling may not work on these same principles. Therefore, if you are involved in another treatment program that is not specifically integrated with this one, you should wait until that program is finished before starting this one. Different programs can provide mixed messages about what you should be doing to manage your symptoms. If you are seeing a therapist or receiving counseling for a totally different reason (for example, marital counseling, or a meditation group), it should be possible to do both at the same time. If you have questions about whether any treatment you are receiving is compatible with this program, you could ask your providers to be in contact with each other.

If you are currently taking medication for your symptoms, continue to take it throughout this program. Keep in mind that certain medications are designed to dampen your emotions, however, including common prescriptions like Xanax, Ativan, or Klonopin. If you have questions about your medications and their compatibility with this treatment, you should consult your therapist, primary care doctor, and/or psychiatrist.

CHAPTER 3

Recording Your Experiences: Eating, Depression, and Anxiety (EDA)

GOALS

- Learn the importance of recordkeeping.
- Introduce you to the Eating, Depression, and Anxiety (EDA) rating scale.
- Introduce you to Form 3.1: Eating, Depression, and Anxiety (EDA).
- Learn how to monitor your experiences for 1 week.

Why take the time to record?

There are many reasons why it is important to keep records of your experiences on a regular, ongoing basis. First, eating disorders, anxiety, mood difficulties, or other uncomfortable emotional experiences typically feel out of your control, as if they have a life of their own. You may 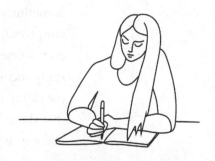 sometimes feel as if you are a victim of your own uncomfortable or distressing experiences. Learning to be an *observer* of your own experience is a first step toward gaining control. You will be learning specific skills to help you understand your emotional experiences in later chapters, but even the simple act of recording your experiences helps you begin to understand them. Through recordkeeping, you will learn to observe when, where, and under what circumstances eating issues and other emotional experiences occur.

Second, you will learn to recognize how what you think, what you feel, and what you do can contribute to these experiences. It is often very difficult to remember everything we were thinking, feeling in our bodies, and doing when an uncomfortable emotional experience occurred—particularly later in a therapy session. If we write these things down closer to the event, we have much more information to recognize and identify different parts of our experience.

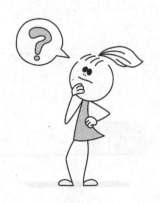

Third, our memories are often general and colored by how we are feeling in the moment. If we were asked to describe the past week, we might say it was "bad," whereas if someone was asking you at different times of each day how you are feeling, it might turn out that on two specific times during the week, you were feeling relatively good. The difficult times are so intense that naturally we focus on them, and it can be hard to remember when you weren't feeling that way. It is useful to also focus on what may contribute to days or times that are better. It is important to realize that negative judgments—such as *the week has been bad*—may be contributing to your overall feelings of anxiety or depression. If you are able to notice that your mood state actually fluctuates, you may be able to develop a more positive sense of yourself and your emotional state.

Sometimes people are concerned that continually recording their eating symptoms, their levels of anxiety, and their mood will make them feel even worse. You might feel concerned about this if you find yourself already focusing a lot on your eating or your distress, and worrying about the eating symptoms and distress itself. It is important to realize, however, that there is a difference between observing your experiences in a *subjective* way as opposed to an *objective* way.

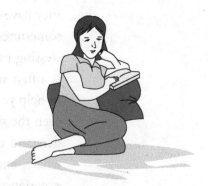

Subjective monitoring means just thinking about or talking about how bad you feel, how out of control you feel, how much your problems bother you, how much they get in the way of your life, or how helpless and overwhelmed you feel about them. You probably already do a lot of subjective monitoring, and you might already be trying to stop thinking about these things so much because it makes you feel worse. It is a little like being inside the middle of a storm and trying to describe how scared you are.

Objective monitoring, which we are asking you to try here, is quite different. Objective monitoring means recording different aspects of your problems in a more "scientific" way. Using a storm analogy, it would be more like taking measurements of the rainfall, changes in the wind speed, and variation of light and dark. In this program you will learn to record things such as how many times in a day or a week you did a certain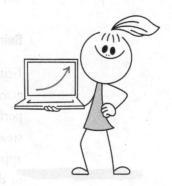

thing or felt a certain way; what was happening right before that; and how you responded in your thoughts, feelings, and behavior. In other words, you will focus on recording facts and observations, and not focus on judgments of yourself or evaluations of how difficult it was (though we care about these things as well!).

At first, it may be difficult to switch from subjective to objective monitoring, and as you start to use the records, you may notice an increase in distress because you are still focusing in the old, subjective way. However, with practice, you will begin to find that switching into the objective mode becomes easier and easier. Let's review the benefits of ongoing monitoring and recording:

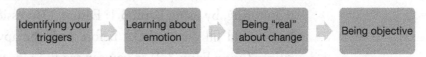

To help you do this, we have included very specific forms in this program that are designed to record very specific objective information.

Identifying your triggers

Identifying your triggers means being able to identify specific triggers of episodes of eating symptoms, anxiety, depression, and other distressing emotional experiences. Knowledge of these triggers and situations will lessen your sense of being out of control of your emotional experiences. It is easy to lose track of the specifics—they can be subtle, and you can start to respond out of habit, without even knowing what you are responding to. Recordkeeping will help you figure this out.

Learning about emotions

Learning about emotions means learning to identify objective, specific aspects of your eating and emotions. These include your behaviors, physical feelings, and thoughts.

Being "real" about change

Being real about change means learning to evaluate the success of your attempts to change. Remember, when you are depressed and anxious, or perfectionistic and self-critical, it is easy to dismiss gains and focus instead on how terrible things are. Objective monitoring will help you to appreciate your progress and gains. When an episode of eating symptoms or distress makes you feel as if you have failed or taken a step back, the records will show the changes that you've made, so that the one incident does not overshadow your progress.

Objectivity

Objectivity means learning to become an objective observer of yourself so that you can begin to stand outside the storm. This is an important step in your progress. It's a good idea to keep all your forms so you can look back from time to time.

Eating, Depression, and Anxiety (EDA) form

This session is to help you understand and make the best use of your self-monitoring, by using Form 3.1: Eating, Depression, and Anxiety (EDA). You should fill out an EDA before each therapy session and graph the ratings (using Form 3.2) so you can see and reflect on the patterns of your symptoms over time.

The EDA is like an emotional snapshot of your day. If we could represent your emotional experience of that day in one snapshot, this is what the EDA tries to do. Another way to think of this is like you are a scientist, collecting data on what you observe to be happening on any given

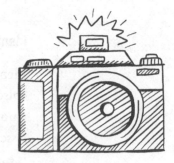

day—only in this scenario you are not only the scientist but also the subject! In this session, we will discuss in detail why the EDA is important, but before we do that it may be useful for us to actually do one together. The reason why it's important will make more sense when you understand the nuts and bolts of how to use it.

In-Session Exercise 3.1
EDA

You will need the following items to complete this activity:

- Form 3.1: Eating, Depression, and Anxiety (EDA). This questionnaire can be found near the end of this chapter.
- The matching EDA Graph (Form 3.2), which also appears at the end of this chapter
- Highlighters or colored markers

When you are ready, start with Steps 1 and 2 pictured in the process below, but don't go on to Step 3 just yet:

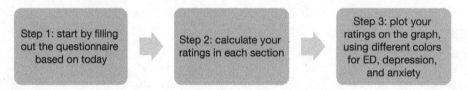

As you probably noticed, there are sections for eating disorder, depression, and anxiety scores. Each section has a question asking how intense your symptoms are, and a question asking how much those symptoms have made it difficult to function. Each score can range from 0 (meaning no symptoms or interference at all) to 8 (meaning the most intense symptoms possible and complete inability to function due to those symptoms). A score of 4 would be midway between those poles.

In Step 3, you are going to learn how to graph these scores. You will begin graphing for homework. Figure 3.1 shows an example graph of the first 5 days of someone's treatment.

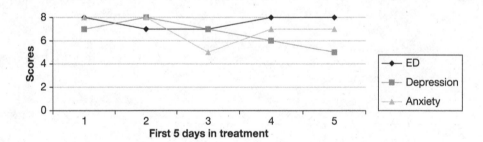

Figure 3.1:

Learning to Plot Your Scores on the EDA Graph

What do the scores mean?

Tracking your emotions is the activity of regularly observing your emotions at regular intervals—it could be every day, every time you have a therapy session, or every week—and monitoring how they peak and fall and regulate based on many factors, such as your inner experiences, your behavior, and things that happen to you. Imagine that you have graphed the score of your eating disorder symptoms over time, and the graph looks like the simple one shown in Figure 3.2.

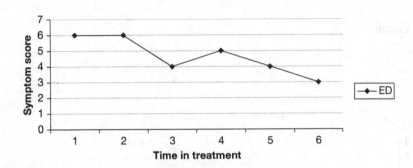

Figure 3.2:

Example ED Graph

A deeper understanding of the EDA

Now we are going to look at a little more complicated graph. This is a client's graph showing all three parts of the EDA tracked over most of the time that this client (who was filling out her EDA daily) was in treatment. In total, she tracked just over 12½ weeks of treatment at multiple levels of care, and we are going to look at two different snapshots of her journey to help us understand the EDA in a deeper way. Figure 3.3 shows her first month of treatment, and Figure 3.4 shows weeks 7 to 10. After about 1 month, this client transitioned from residential to day treatment, and toward the end of the second month she moved to a different state. It is worth noting that after 2 weeks of residential treatment, she was no longer reporting any behavioral symptoms, but continued to experience urges at varying intensities. We are going to trace over each of the lines with a different color. This will make the eating disorder, depression, and anxiety lines really pop out while we're talking about what her scores mean.

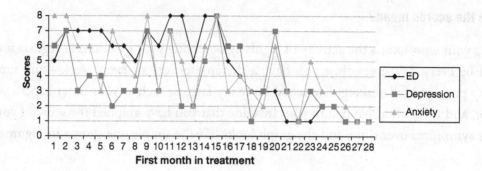

Figure 3.3:

Example EDA Graph

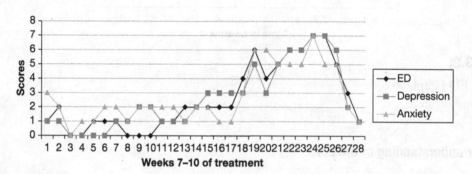

Figure 3.4:

Example EDA Graph

28

Many of the forms and worksheets will need to be filled out more than once. We are including one blank copy of every worksheet and form for you. For those items that you will need more than once, your therapist will provide additional copies, or you can download blank copies yourself from the TreatmentsThatWork™ website at www.oxfordclinicalpsych.com/UTforEDs.

- Fill out Form 3.1: Eating, Depression, and Anxiety (EDA).
- Plot scores on Form 3.2: EDA Graph.
- Read Chapter 4 and preview the exercises.

Eating, Depression, and Anxiety (EDA)

1. How intense or severe were your urges to engage in eating disorder (ED) symptoms today?

0 = *None*: ED urges absent or barely noticeable.

1 = *Mild*: Urges at a low level. It was possible to not engage in ED symptoms.

2 = *Moderate*: ED urges were distressing at times. I had ED symptoms at points during the day.

3 = *Severe*: ED urges were intense much of the time. I had ED symptoms during most of the day.

4 = *Extreme*: ED urges were overwhelming. I thought about little else outside of ED symptoms.

2. How much did your ED interfere with your ability to do the things you needed to do in the past day?

0 = *None*: No interference from my ED symptoms.

1 = *Mild*: My ED has caused some interference. Things are harder, but I am getting them done.

2 = *Moderate*: My ED definitely interferes. I'm not doing all the things I would normally do.

3 = *Severe*: My ability to function has seriously suffered due to my ED.

4 = *Extreme*: My ED has become incapacitating. I am unable to complete important tasks.

SUM OF #1 + #2: _____ *Plot this number as a circle on your graph.*

3. In the past day, when you have felt depressed, how intense or severe was your depression?

0 = *Little or None*: Depression was absent or barely noticeable.

1 = *Mild*: Depression was at a low level.

2 = *Moderate*: Depression was intense at times.

3 = *Severe*: Depression was intense much of the time.

4 = *Extreme*: Depression was overwhelming.

4. In the past day, how much did depression interfere with your ability to do things you needed to do?

0 = *None*: No interference from depression.

1 = *Mild*: Depression has caused some interference. Things are harder, but I am getting them done.

2 = *Moderate*: Depression definitely interfering. I'm not doing all the things I would normally do.

3 = *Severe*: My ability to function has seriously suffered due to my depression.

4 = *Extreme*: My depression has become incapacitating. I am unable to complete important tasks.

SUM OF #3 + #4 _____ *Plot this number as a square on your graph.*

5. In the past day, when you have felt anxious, how intense or severe was your anxiety?

0 = *None*: Anxiety was absent or barely noticeable.

1 = *Mild*: Anxiety was at a low. It was possible to relax when I tried.

2 = *Moderate*: Anxiety was distressing at times. It was hard to relax or concentrate, but I could do it.

3 = *Severe*: Anxiety was intense much of the time. It was very difficult to relax or focus.

4 = *Extreme*: Anxiety was overwhelming. It was impossible to relax at all.

6. How much did your anxiety interfere with your ability to do things you needed to do in the past day?

0 = *None*: No interference from anxiety.

1 = *Mild*: My depression has caused some interference. Things are hard, but I'm getting them done.

2 = *Moderate*: My anxiety definitely interferes. I'm not doing all the things I would normally do.

3 = *Severe*: My ability to function has seriously suffered due to my anxiety.

4 = *Extreme*: My anxiety has become incapacitating. I am unable to complete important tasks.

SUM OF #5 + #6 _____ *Plot this number as a triangle on your graph.*

Form 3.2
EDA Graph

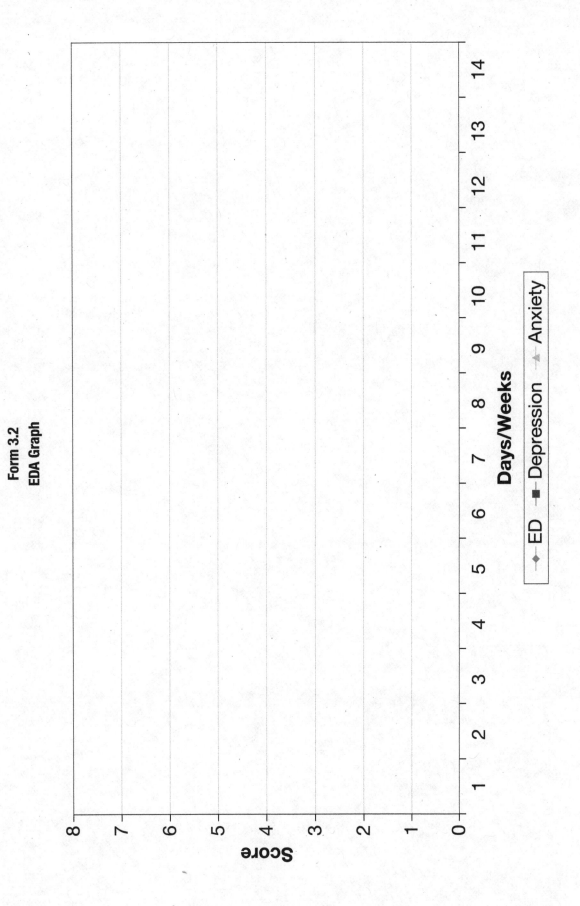

Score

Days/Weeks

◆ ED ■ Depression ▲ Anxiety

Motivation and Goals

Motivation and Regular Eating

GOALS

- Discuss the importance of motivation.
- Explore the costs and benefits of changing.
- Explore the costs and benefits of remaining the same.
- Set specific goals you hope to achieve during treatment.
- Set manageable steps to reach treatment goals.

HOMEWORK REVIEW

- Fill out Form 3.1: Eating, Depression, and Anxiety (EDA).
- Plot scores on Form 3.2: EDA Graph.
- Read Chapter 4 and preview the exercises.

Motivation

It is important to think about *why* you want to change and your reasons for doing the work that change requires. Two things will strongly influence your treatment outcome:

- Treatment engagement: How engaged you are in treatment is *directly* related to how well you respond to treatment. *In other words, the more you engage in treatment, the better the outcome.*

- Treatment commitment: How motivated and committed you are to the treatment process is also directly related to how well you respond to treatment. *The more reasons you have to keep going, and the more you pay attention to these reasons, the more motivated you are.*

You have likely been through a lot to get to the point of needing treatment. **So, your job is to make the *most* of your treatment experience to get the best result you can get**. As with most things in life, you get out only as much as you put in. In treatment this means reading and thinking about the material, participating in self-reflection in sessions, and doing the homework exercises. But motivation is complicated!

Motivation can be like a roller coaster

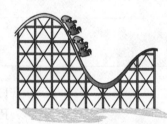

Some days your motivation will be high and doing your treatment will be easier. However, some days it might be more difficult to get yourself to complete the homework or exercises. It is on these days that it is most important to push yourself.

Things outside of you can affect your motivation

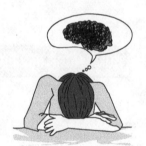

Increased stresses, feeling tired or sick, or having a busy week can all reduce your motivation for engaging in treatment. Recognizing that external factors can affect your motivation is important.

Ambivalence is OK

There will be times that you might even feel like you no longer want to change, or that change is not worth the time and effort. This is a natural part of the change process. It is important to allow yourself to have these moments.

In-Session Exercise 4.1
Q&A on Achieving Difficult Things

Please think of something in the past that you achieved that was really difficult (such as "I completed my undergraduate degree" or "I made the team"). What about that was hard? What helped you to stay motivated? Write your answers to these questions below.

Past achievement: _____

What about that was hard?_____

What helped you to stay motivated?_____

In-Session Exercise 4.2
Decisional Balance Activity

Most people at this point in treatment have mixed feelings about their eating disorder, other emotional problems, and pursuing recovery. At times you might feel confused or overwhelmed by these conflicting feelings and give up thinking about them altogether. Thinking through the good reasons to change and the strong reasons NOT to change can help the process feel more manageable. Start by identifying the problem areas—perhaps based on your diagnostic information, or perhaps just whatever you struggle with—that you came to treatment for help with. These should be things you would be interested in changing.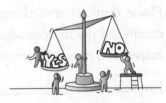

Examples might be "eating disorder," "social isolation," "OCD," or "body image problems." Write as few or as many as you like:

1._____

2._____

Others:_____

_____

_____

For each of these areas, we are going to identify key pros and cons of change. There are blank copies of some of the Chapter 4 worksheets later in this chapter.

In-Session Exercise 4.3
Decisional Balance Exercise

People want to change because they don't want to keep feeling this way, and they don't want to continue to be limited in their lives. Think about all the ways your symptoms have gotten in the way of living the life you want. Do you have values, goals, or qualities that have been compromised by the eating disorder, depression, or anxiety? If things stay the same, how will things look a year from now? What wouldn't you like about that? How has your life changed since you became this way—what would you like to have back?

Problem area: _____

Cons/Costs *Why don't you want to change?* *Why do you want to stay the same?*	Pros/Benefits *Why do you want to change?* *Why don't you want to stay the same?*

In-Session Exercise 4.4
Setting Goals Activity

This worksheet can be difficult. It might feel like the steps necessary to meeting your goal are not manageable, or it is hard to see yourself actually doing some of these things. These are common feelings!

As you go through treatment, you will learn skills that will help to make the emotions more manageable, although it is hard to believe this 100 percent now. Keep in mind that the goal of this section is to come up with specific behaviors that can be completed in a specific timeframe, such as "Eat lunch" as opposed to "Recover from my eating disorder."

Research shows that *regular eating* is an important part of recovery. Most individuals with eating disorders do not eat regularly—meaning eating three meals and two or three snacks, or eating roughly every 3 to 4 hours throughout the day. One important goal is regular eating. However, this can be a very difficult goal to achieve! To make it more manageable, one of the goals for each session at the beginning of treatment will be taking steps toward that goal. We will address regular eating first, and set more personalized goals next.

One of my goals for early treatment is:

<u>Regular eating</u>

Making it more concrete

Now, we are going to make this goal more concrete. We have set some guidelines, and you can identify what other things you would be doing or not doing.

THINGS I WANT TO DO (regular eating):

<u>Eating three meals and two or three snacks per day</u>

<u>Eating roughly every 3–4 hours and not eating between these times</u>

<u>Eating enough to maintain a healthy weight for my body</u>

THINGS I WANT TO STOP DOING (for example, dieting/restricting, binge eating, grazing, or compensatory behaviors such as purging by vomiting, laxative abuse, or compulsive exercise):

_____

_____

In-Session Exercise 4.5
Introduction to "Taking the Necessary Steps"

Next, think about some small steps that you can take toward reaching the specific treatment goal you have recorded earlier in this form. These steps should take anywhere from a few days to a week to achieve. It can be helpful to work backward from your goal to help identify specific steps. Use the behaviors listed earlier in this form to help come up with specific steps. If you are working with a nutritionist/dietitian, you may be setting goals in those sessions as well. This work can support those goals or add to them.

Are there any steps you can be trying to take between now and your next session of therapy?

Step 1: _Write down my eating, compensatory behaviors, and notes in self-monitoring log_

Step 2: _____

Step 3: _____

Step 4: _____

One personal goal for treatment is:

_____

Making it more concrete

What would it look like once you have achieved this goal? What concrete things would you be doing, or not doing? What behaviors would you be engaging in, or *not* engaging in?

_____

_____

_____

Conclusion

It is important to have goals for change, meaning something in the future that we want, or that we don't want. These can include more immediate things such as "practicing homework exercises tonight" or more distant things such as "making more friends" and "feeling happier." **The more specific and concrete our goal is, the more likely we will be successful.** For example, the goal of "practicing relaxation exercises tonight" is much more likely to lead to successful behavioral change than the goal of "being a relaxed person." Take a look at Box 4.1: Sample Completed "Taking the Necessary Steps" Worksheet on p. 44. How did this person do at being realistic, concrete, and achievable?

Homework

Many of the forms and worksheets will need to be filled out more than once. We are including one blank copy of every worksheet and form for you. For those items that you will need more than once, your therapist will provide additional copies, or you can download blank copies yourself from the TreatmentsThatWork™ website at www.oxfordclinicalpsych.com/UTforEDs.

- Fill out Form 3.1: Eating, Depression, and Anxiety (EDA).
- Plot scores on Form 3.2: EDA Graph.
- Fill out Form 4.1: Regular Eating Food Log. You and your therapist should discuss if it is a good idea to fill out Form 4.1 each day. We do recommend using the actual form, which as noted earlier is available to download, particularly if you do not eat regularly or experience binge eating and/or compensatory behaviors. The form has a column labeled "B?" where you can put a mark in the column if an eating event was a binge episode. It also has a column labeled "CB?" where you can put a mark if you purged by vomiting, used laxatives, or used diuretics as a compensatory behavior. The form should not be used to record calories or measurements, just general descriptions of the food and the amount, along with the other information listed.
- Review Box 4.1: Sample Completed "Taking the Necessary Steps" Worksheet, and then fill out Worksheet 4.1: "Taking the Necessary Steps" Homework Sheet for yourself.
- Read Chapter 5 and preview the exercises.

Form 4.1
Regular Eating Food Log

This is a format for keeping a food log on a daily basis. You should fill out one for each day. It is important NOT to record calories. Although your mind may have habits, it is important to stop writing down calories and start writing down other information, with the goal of eventually eating three meals and two or three snacks without eating between. Your nutrition team may have other goals and techniques as well. Please share this with them.

Time	Foods	Place	B?	CB?	Emotions, Thoughts, Physical Sensations

Box 4.1
Sample Completed "Taking the Necessary Steps" Worksheet

Your treatment goal that you will begin working toward within the next 24 hours:

To do 3 snacks daily (at roughly 10 a.m., 3 p.m., and 9 p.m.) by the end of this week

Making it more concrete

Now, let's take a moment to make this goal more concrete. What would it look like once you have achieved this goal? What things would you be doing, or not doing? What behaviors would you be engaging in? What behaviors would you _not_ be engaging in? Try to be as concrete as possible here.

If I achieved the goal, then I would be completing 100% of these snacks. I would not be drinking meal replacement shakes, and instead would be eating actual "snacky foods" that have nutritional value. I would also be on track with my weight goals. I would be eating at an even pace. I would not be selecting "low-cal" or "diet" options unless my dietitian tells me I can. I would also decrease my use of food rituals like eating food in a certain order, or excessively wiping my fingers on my napkin. I would also be finishing my meals and completing my Food Log.

Taking the necessary steps

Next, think about some small manageable steps that you can take toward reaching the specific treatment goals you've listed earlier in this form. These steps should take anywhere from a few days or a week up to a month to achieve. What steps will you need to take? It can be helpful to work backward from your goal to help identify specific steps you will need to take to get there. Use the behaviors you listed earlier in this form to help come up with your steps to achieving your treatment goal.

Step 1:

Today and moving forward I will plan my snack choices for the next day, and pack them into a cooler or lunch bag so that I can take them with me.

Step 2:

I will plan to eat my meals at regular times, so that I don't run into the problem of having had a "late lunch" and then skipping my mid-afternoon snack.

Step 3:

Even if I don't feel hungry at snack time, I will still eat the recommended snack. I will remind myself that my body is still adjusting to regular eating, and I will journal about my feelings on this.

Step 4:

Share this goal with my therapist and dietitian so they know what I am trying to do. I will ask them to give me feedback on my progress, to see if there are any behaviors I need to adjust.

Worksheet 4.1
"Taking the Necessary Steps" Homework Sheet

This worksheet can be difficult. It might feel like the steps necessary to meeting your goal are not manageable, or it may be hard to see yourself actually doing some of these things. These are common feelings! When completing this worksheet, ask yourself whether the steps you are writing down are specific behaviors that can be completed in a limited time period, not whether you believe you are capable of completing them currently.

As you go through treatment, you will learn skills that will be helpful and will ultimately make the emotions begin to feel more manageable, although it is hard to believe this 100 percent now. Keep in mind that the goal of this section is to come up with specific behaviors that can be completed in a specific timeframe, such as "Eat my whole lunch," as opposed to "Recover from my eating disorder."

One goal for treatment is:

_____

Making it more concrete

Now, let's take a moment to make this goal more concrete. What would it look like once you have achieved this goal? What things would you be doing, or not doing? What behaviors would you be engaging in? What behaviors would you *not* be engaging in? Try to be as concrete as possible here.

_____

_____

Taking the necessary steps

Next, think about some small steps that you can take toward reaching the specific treatment goal you have recorded earlier in this form. These steps should take anywhere from a few days or a week up to a month to achieve, but there is a line to think about whether there is anything you can do in the next 24 hours to take a step along this path. It can be helpful to work backward from your goal to help identify specific steps. Use the behaviors listed earlier in this form to help come up with specific steps.

Are there any steps you can be trying to take between now and your next session of therapy?

Step 1:_____

Step 2:_____

Step 3:_____

Step 4:_____

Another goal for treatment is:

_____

Making it more concrete

Take a moment to make this goal more concrete. What would it look like once you have achieved this goal? What things would you be doing, or not doing? What behaviors would you be engaging in or *not* engaging in? Again, being as concrete as possible here, try to list specific behaviors.

_____

Taking the necessary steps

Next, think about some small manageable steps that you can take towards reaching the specific treatment goals you've listed earlier in this form. These steps should take anywhere from a few days or a week up to a month to achieve. What steps will you need to take? It can be helpful to work backward from your goal to help identify specific steps you will need to take to get there. Use the behaviors you listed earlier in this form to help come up with your steps to achieving your treatment goal.

Are there any steps you can be trying to take in the next 24 hours?

Step 1:_____

Step 2:_____

Step 3:_____

Step 4:_____

GOALS

- Describe regular eating.
- Discuss the importance of regular eating.
- Explore what regular eating would look like for you.
- Brainstorm ideas for overcoming obstacles to regular eating.

HOMEWORK REVIEW

- Fill out Form 3.1: Eating, Depression, and Anxiety (EDA).
- Plot scores on Form 3.2: EDA Graph.
- Fill out Form 4.1: Regular Eating Food Log. You and your therapist should discuss if it is a good idea to fill out Form 4.1 each day. We do recommend using the actual form, which is available to download, particularly if you do not eat regularly or experience binge eating and/or compensatory behaviors. The form has a column labeled "B?" where you can put a mark in the column if an eating event involved loss of control over eating, in which case it was a binge episode. It also has a column labeled "CB?" where you can put a mark if you purged by vomiting, used laxatives, exercised, fasted, or used diuretics specifically as a compensatory behavior. The form should not be used to record calories or measurements, just general descriptions of the food and the amount, along with the other information listed.

- Review Figure 4.1: Sample Completed "Taking the Necessary Steps" Worksheet, and then fill out Worksheet 4.1: "Taking the Necessary Steps" Homework Sheet for yourself.
- Read Chapter 5 and preview the exercises.

How did it go trying to record your eating and emotional experiences in the food log? How did your other homework go? The first week that you record your eating, you might learn a lot about your eating patterns overall, including events and situations that trigger certain behaviors. We are going to take the first part of the session to discuss what you have noticed.

Regular eating

At this point in treatment, it is a goal to start eating regularly, which means eating three "meals" and two or three "snacks" per day. If you are not a person who eats regularly, this may be very hard! Therefore, the first step of this goal is just to eat on a schedule, without a goal about what makes up each meal and snack. You should choose what- ever foods you think you can eat, in order to start eating at the right times of day. Based on when you get up and when you go to bed, this means that you will eat roughly every 3 to 4 hours. Here are some guidelines:

- Never go more than 4 hours without eating.
- Time your eating so that there are at least 2 hours between events.
- Three snacks are ideal if you have 4 or more hours between breakfast and lunch and 3 or more hours between dinner and bedtime. If breakfast and lunch are much closer together, then plan two snacks. If you stay up much later following dinner, you may need an additional snack at night.

Figure 5.1 is an example of how someone who has *been restricting* and *gets up early* might take one step closer toward regular eating. This is not an example of a "good" diet overall—please don't judge the example or yourself based on the example. It probably doesn't include enough nutrients for most people.

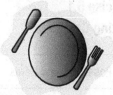

8 am "Breakfast"	2 boiled eggs
10 am "Snack"	A piece of fruit
12 pm "Lunch"	A salad with some protein
3 pm "Snack"	A small granola bar
7 pm "Dinner"	A piece of chicken, a lot of vegetables,
10 pm "Snack"	2 handfuls of dried berries

Figure 5.1:

Example Regular Eating Schedule

Figure 5.2 is also an example of regular eating.

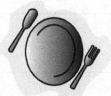

10 am "Breakfast"	Eggs, toast, home-fries, fruit salad
1 pm "Lunch"	Turkey sub, veggies and mayo, side s：
4 pm "Snack"	Vegetables, pita, hummus, falafel
7 pm "Dinner"	Chickpea stew, rice, apple
8:30 "Snack"	Ice cream
11:00"Snack"	Bowl of cereal with milk

Figure 5.2:

Example Regular Eating Schedule

Once again, we are not providing examples of good or bad eating from a nutritional perspective. We are trying to show you how two very different days of food can both be good examples of "regular eating," meaning three meals and two or three snacks, spread out over the day, about every 2 to 4 hours.

Using In-Session Exercise 5.1, let's generate roughly the right times for you to be eating, and then talk about a few options for each of those times.

In-Session Exercise 5.1
Personal Regular Eating Calendar

Meal	Time	Possible Food Items
Breakfast		
Snack		
Lunch		
Snack		
Dinner		
Snack		

YOU pick what YOU can do in order to keep going. If you eat something that is unplanned, then immediately try to get back on schedule by eating the next meal/snack, even if you aren't hungry.

I definitely can't eat that amount of food. If I could eat that regularly, I wouldn't have an eating disorder! How am I supposed to do this?

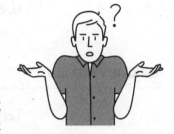

You are just going to start trying and writing down when it works and when it doesn't work in your log, and we are going to problem-solve together. There is no expectation that you will be able to do this perfectly right away!

This is not the same as what is in the meal plan I got from my nutritionist. Which one should I do?

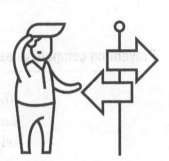

Your nutritionist has more responsibility for helping you plan *what* you eat. This form is more about *when* you eat. Your meal plan is also a goal that you are working toward, and eating regularly is a good first step. We want you to have flexibility in what you eat over time, but the first way to start with that is to eat according to the clock, and we have to be realistic about what you can commit to—instead of setting goals that are unrealistic and then being disappointed when they are too hard. Please bring your food log to show your nutritionist, so that every member of your team can help out.

Eating according to the clock is not how people eat in real life. If I have just eaten a few hours earlier, or overeaten, I might not be hungry for the next snack or meal. Aren't people supposed to eat when they are hungry?

That is true. Once again, in real life, people who don't have eating disorders have flexibility in what they eat. Sometimes they eat because hunger tells them to. Sometimes they actually eat when they aren't hungry—because it is social, or because they know some time is going to go by later when it will be hard to get food. Your hunger cues may also be affected negatively by your experience of an eating disorder. Two ways to "reset" your hunger cues appropriately are first to eat regularly, and then to work toward eating what your body needs in terms of energy and nutrients, including having the flexibility to eat anything. Once those goals are achieved, then eating according to what your body tells you and what is available to you—that is, eating "intuitively"—is possible and healthy.

Tackling obstacles

Let's look ahead at the next set of days between now and when we meet again, and think about what events, each day, could possibly get in the way of the plan. Use Worksheet 5.1: Weekly Obstacle Sheet to generate ideas for how to tackle obstacles this week.

Preventing compulsive eating

The first part of eating regularly is to put the eating events in place on the right schedule. The other part of eating regularly is not to eat in between those times. Of course, it is not a disaster to eat, but for the time being you want to have some practice eating at certain times (which is a challenge in one way) and not eating at other times (which is a challenge in another way).

If you have eaten according to the schedule, and eaten enough food to provide energy for your body, then some of the urges that you have to eat between meals and snacks, or to eat more than you have planned, will likely be due to habitual thoughts, behaviors, and physical sensations. These are the components of emotional experi-

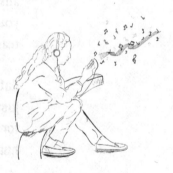

ence as well. If you have urges to eat between regular eating events or to eat more than you have planned, it is a good idea to record this information on Form 4.1: Regular Eating Food Log. Try not to act on the feelings (the urges to eat) immediately, and take some time to write them down. Try to wait a little while to see if the feelings pass. If it would help to take a walk, or have a conversation, or listen to some music, these are good ways to pass the time. Do try to make some notes about what was going on and whether you were able to wait out the urge.

One important thing we will emphasize throughout the program is that *emotions always pass*. They also often come back again. But if you can break the chain between emotions (thoughts, physical sensations, and urges/behaviors) and behaviors that are part of your emotional disorder, you can develop new flexibility and transform your emotional experience.

Use Worksheet 5.2: Activities to Delay Compulsive Eating to list some activities you might do in situations to delay acting on the urge to eat in problematic ways. Start generating some ideas now, and your therapist can help add to the list in session.

Homework

Many of the forms and worksheets will need to be filled out more than once. We are including one blank copy of every worksheet and form for you. For those items that you will need more than once, your therapist will provide additional copies, or you can download blank copies yourself from the TreatmentsThatWork™ website at www.oxfordclinicalpsych.com/UTforEDs.

- Fill out Form 3.1: Eating, Depression, and Anxiety (EDA).
- Plot scores on Form 3.2: EDA Graph.
- Fill out Form 4.1: Regular Eating Food Log.
- Fill out Worksheet 5.1: Weekly Obstacle Sheet and Worksheet 5.2: Activities to Delay Compulsive Eating.
- Read Chapter 6 and preview the exercises.

Worksheet 5.1
Weekly Obstacle Sheet

List the days of the week between now and your next session across the top of the chart. Then make notes about possible obstacles to regular eating, and solutions.

	Tomorrow _____	_____	_____	_____	_____
Breakfast	Obstacle? Y / N If Y, what? Solution?	Obstacle? Y / N If Y, what? Solution?	Obstacle? Y / N If Y, what? Solution?	Obstacle? Y / N If Y, what? Solution?	Obstacle? Y / N If Y, what? Solution?
Snack	Obstacle? Y / N If Y, what? Solution?	Obstacle? Y / N If Y, what? Solution?	Obstacle? Y / N If Y, what? Solution?	Obstacle? Y / N If Y, what? Solution?	Obstacle? Y / N If Y, what? Solution?
Lunch	Obstacle? Y / N If Y, what? Solution?	Obstacle? Y / N If Y, what? Solution?	Obstacle? Y / N If Y, what? Solution?	Obstacle? Y / N If Y, what? Solution?	Obstacle? Y / N If Y, what? Solution?
Snack	Obstacle? Y / N If Y, what? Solution?	Obstacle? Y / N If Y, what? Solution?	Obstacle? Y / N If Y, what? Solution?	Obstacle? Y / N If Y, what? Solution?	Obstacle? Y / N If Y, what? Solution?
Dinner	Obstacle? Y / N If Y, what? Solution?	Obstacle? Y / N If Y, what? Solution?	Obstacle? Y / N If Y, what? Solution?	Obstacle? Y / N If Y, what? Solution?	Obstacle? Y / N If Y, what? Solution?
Snack	Obstacle? Y / N If Y, what? Solution?	Obstacle? Y / N If Y, what? Solution?	Obstacle? Y / N If Y, what? Solution?	Obstacle? Y / N If Y, what? Solution?	Obstacle? Y / N If Y, what? Solution?

Worksheet 5.2
Activities to Delay Compulsive Eating

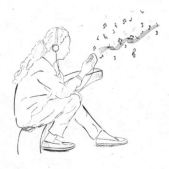

In order to stop automatic chains of behavior and to take time to reflect on your emotions, it is good to have some immediate ideas of alternative activities right at hand. You might want to post your list somewhere (in your phone, on the wall) where you can see it to remind you when your mind is consumed with acting on your impulses. If you are able to take some time to delay acting on the urge, you may notice that the urge changes or that you learn something about what you were feeling and thinking in the moment (to write in your food log!).

Alternative activities should be pleasant and easy to do in the moment. They should basically help you to tolerate your emotions and urges without punishing yourself for your emotions and urges.

Examples:

Walking	Listening to music	Taking a shower	Meditating	Writing in a journal or food log
Calling someone	Internet shopping	Watching a show	Reading a book	Walking to buy a magazine
Lighting a candle	Playing Jenga	Listening to a podcast	Being outside	Solo games like Sudoku

Everyone's list is going to be personal and different. Try to generate 5 to 10 personal, specific things (for example, "Walking to the library and back while listening to my favorite album" or "Calling my mom and just talking about how the day went" or "Reading my novel").

Write your list here:

1.

2.

3.

4.

5.

6.

7.

8.

9.

10.

Understanding Emotion

The Natural Function of Emotions

CHAPTER 6   The Natural Function of Emotions

GOAL

- Understand the natural and adaptive function (the evolutionary purpose) of each emotion.

HOMEWORK REVIEW

- Fill out Form 3.1: Eating, Depression, and Anxiety (EDA).
- Plot scores on Form 3.2: EDA Graph.
- Fill out Form 4.1: Regular Eating Food Log.
- Fill out Worksheet 5.1: Weekly Obstacle Sheet and Worksheet 5.2: Activities to Delay Compulsive Eating.
- Read Chapter 6 and preview the exercises.

Functions of emotions

As illustrated in Figure 6.1, emotions are crucial to human psychology, survival, and our day-to-day experience.

Why do we focus so much on emotions? Because *the symptoms of eating disorders, anxiety, and depression come from difficulties with coping with uncomfortable or distressing emotional experiences.*

You may have a lot of different perspectives on your emotions. The first step is to understand how all the emotions, even the ones we don't like, could be adaptive, and all help human beings to function when they are working correctly. You may feel like:

- I don't have a problem with emotions; I have a problem with (conflict, eating, my body, other people, etc.).
- My emotions are the problem, because they are too intense.

All of these observations are legitimate and important, and we will fully deal with them later. For now, for the purposes of this treatment, we practice thinking of all the emotions as being useful or adaptive, even though some emotions are easier and some are more difficult to tolerate.

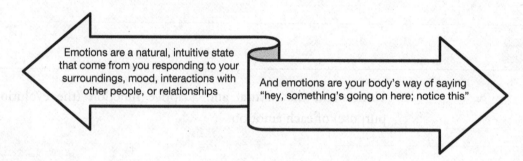

Figure 6.1:
How We Understand Emotions

In-Session Exercise 6.1
Trying On Emotions

Fear

Fear is crucial to our survival. Sometimes it is important to react quickly to danger with a "fight or flight" response.

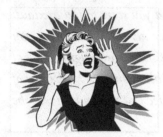

Imagine you are crossing the street with a friend. Suddenly, a car comes screeching and careening straight toward you. Without thinking, you jump onto the sidewalk and pull your friend to safety away from the oncoming car.

So, how was fear helpful in this situation?

- _____
- _____
- _____

Sadness

We often neglect to note the very important function of sadness in our lives. It is a signal to us and to others that something important has changed, requiring some time and attention.

Imagine you find out that a very close friend or family member or a beloved pet has passed away. You will probably feel intense sadness and a great sense of loss. You feel as if you have no energy and it is hard focus on anything else except on your loss. You might feel like sleeping, crying, or staying home, and possibly talking about the person who you lost with people you love.

What could be useful about being sad in this situation?

- _____
- _____
- _____

Anxiety

Anxiety serves a very important function! It is a *future-oriented* state; it has to do with getting ready to cope with future events. When we feel anxious, our bodies and minds go into a state of alertness and "preparation" so that we aren't caught off guard if something bad happens.

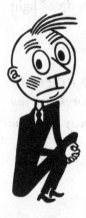

Imagine that you have a presentation coming up, which is important for your job or grade. You think about it often as the date approaches and you start to feel anxious. You do research on the topic, and you work late to gather all the information you need. You prepare the presentation and practice it several times. You imagine some of the questions people might ask and write down some possible answers. On the day of the presentation, you get up earlier than usual, put on nice clothes, and review the presentation.

How did anxiety help out in this situation? How was it good?

- _____
- _____
- _____

Anger

Anger is focused on keeping things fair and also on acting to defend your rights, values, and safety. It is the "fight" side of "fight or flight," or the referee in the game of life.

Imagine you discover that the clerk at your local coffee shop has been putting extra charges on your credit card every morning when you go to buy breakfast. You angrily call the store and report the theft to the manager, but the manager says that the clerk has quit and there is no way to get your money back. You demand to speak to the manager's supervisor, and then demand to have the money returned. You say you will go to the police if they cannot help you.

How could anger be helping you here?

- _____
- _____
- _____

Guilt and shame

Guilt and shame are similar but different. Some people say that *guilt* is when you recognize that you have done something specific that is bad, whereas *shame* is an overall feeling that you are a bad person, possibly because of something that you have done, how you see yourself, or how you think someone sees you. Both guilt and shame actually can be adaptive and helpful.

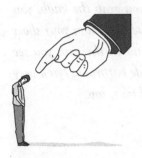

You see there is a voice message on your phone from someone who calls you a lot. You are having a bad day and feel irritated that this person calls so much and often bothers you during busy times. You roll your eyes and delete the message without listening to it. The next day, you realize it was that person's birthday! You forgot to wish them happy birthday and angrily screened the call—and you feel instantly guilty. You realize you were about to do that to your current messages as well, and you feel a little ashamed.

How could guilt and shame be helping you here?

- _____
- _____
- _____

Guilt is a little bit easier because it helps you know you have done something wrong and you want to fix it. Some examples might be making an apology or admitting you were wrong about something. Guilt has a self-correcting function or a reconciliatory function. Shame is meant to serve the same function basically—by noticing there might be something wrong with you--but because shame can make you want to run away, hide, or dissolve into the floorboards, it doesn't always serve that function! One way to think about it is that feeling guilty, feeling ashamed, and feeling embarrassed are all variations of the same point, which is that you have done something that you feel bad about or think others could judge you for. Without those emotions, you wouldn't have a signal about how you are supposed to behave in social groups or relationships.

Disgust

Humans are disgusted by things that may have been contagious at some point in evolution—things that are dirty or smelly, for example, might have germs. Having repulsion for dirty things can protect us.

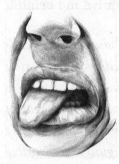

Imagine that you are entering a public bathroom. As you grab the knob, you realize it is a little wet and really sticky. As you enter the bathroom your shoes are also sticking slightly to the floor. Near the toilet and in the sink you see pooled green liquid, partially dried. You realize the whole bathroom has a very sour smell, and you realize that your sticky hands smell sour, too.

How could disgust be helping you here?

■ _____

■ _____

■ _____

As these examples illustrate, emotions serve a very important function in our lives, and at their core, emotions are adaptive experiences. However, as we all know, these emotions can also get in the way, cause a great deal of distress, and cause us to limit the degree to which we are truly living our lives. The truth is, although these emotions are all adaptive in the normal course of anyone's life, sometimes we can experience these emotions as too intense, as too uncontrollable, and as happening in the wrong situation or at the wrong time.

Distress about these emotional experiences plays an important role in keeping symptoms of emotional disorders going. **As you go through this treatment, you will learn how to break cycles of intense, overwhelming emotions.** However, before we can start to understand where emotions become problematic, it is important in the beginning to understand that emotions, even the ones that seem uncomfortable or dysfunctional, can serve an adaptive purpose. They aren't inherently dangerous, and we don't want them to go completely away.

Homework

Many of the forms and worksheets will need to be filled out more than once. We are including one blank copy of every worksheet and form for you. For those items that you will need more than once, your therapist will provide additional copies, or you can download blank copies yourself from the TreatmentsThatWork™ website at www.oxfordclinicalpsych.com/UTforEDs.

- Fill out Form 3.1: Eating, Depression, and Anxiety (EDA).
- Plot scores on Form 3.2: EDA Graph.
- Fill out Form 4.1: Regular Eating Food Log.
- Read and complete Worksheet 6.1: Function of Physical Sensations Homework.
- Read Chapter 7 and preview the exercises.

Worksheet 6.1
Function of Physical Sensations Homework

The physical component of emotions in our bodies can be functional when the emotion is functional. We don't always understand why our bodies feel the way they do, which can be confusing or unpleasant, particularly when the emotion itself seems to be happening at the wrong time or too intensely.

When we have strong emotional reactions, we often have a sympathetic nervous system response. When the sympathetic nervous system kicks into "fight or flight" mode, there is a chain of reactions from the release of hormones like adrenaline. In order to be the best at fighting or the fastest at running away, oxygen and energy need to be distributed around your body quickly.

These hormones cause the following to happen:

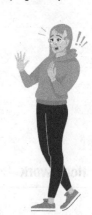

- Your heart beats faster.
- Blood goes to your muscles.
- Muscles tense in readiness for activity.
- Air passages dilate and your breathing speeds up.
- Digestion slows down as energy is diverted for other needs.

Other side effects of these processes can be:

- Palpitations and chest pains
- Sweating
- Dizziness
- Dry mouth
- Trembling
- Tingling
- Muscle tension and stomach cramps
- Feeling faint and sometimes feelings of unreality
- Nausea and stomach pain
- Urge to urinate
- Tightness in the throat and difficulty swallowing

These particular physical reactions are most characteristic of feeling frightened, anxious, angry, and excited. As noted earlier, they are side effects of being ready to fight or flee.

Sadness has its own physiological picture:

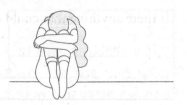

- Crying
- Heaviness
- Fatigue
- Headache
- Stomachache

Researchers think that crying when we are sad is adaptive because it signals to others that we need help. Think of the function of crying for an infant and caregiver—how else would the caregiver know something is needed? In adulthood, people cry when they are in extreme physical or emotional pain, again signaling to others—and to themselves—their helplessness and need for assistance. Some of the physical ways we feel when we are sad or anxious, such as restlessness, are a side effect of our desire to escape from these situations. Over time, we can become anxious and angry about being sad, or sad about being anxious, and these two emotions get intertwined.

Some of the physical experiences of sadness are side effects of crying, such as swollen eyes, headaches, or runny nose. Others are side effects that come from the process of recognizing that something very significant has occurred—either the immediate shock to the system, the onset of crying, or the effort to hold that back.

It is important to understand that these reactions are *normal* and are *functional* for your body in certain situations. They are natural and not dangerous. Though your emotions and the physical component of your emotions may not be helping you right now, it is important to understand and accept the natural and normal functions of your own physical reactions to all emotions. For homework, please identify several intense physical reactions that you have to emotional situations, and see if you can explain how these reactions could be natural and functional, as well as how they may feel dysfunctional or upsetting. Here are two examples:

Example 1

A strong physical sensation with an emotion:

Sometimes when I am talking to a stranger, my stomach growls really loudly. It happens a lot when I really want someone to like me.

How does this physical sensation feel dysfunctional?

I hate it! I am sooooo embarrassed and I worry that the new person is going to think I am crazy. If I want someone to like me, why does my body make me seem like a freak?

How could this physical sensation actually be a normal and natural part of an emotion?

I am nervous and excited, so I guess that's my sympathetic nervous system. My stomach must be reacting by having muscle tension and slowing down digestive processes.

Is there anything that could even be functional about having that emotion?

It is probably a good thing I am excited about this person because otherwise, who cares? Why even try to form a relationship with them? It also could be a good thing to be nervous because it makes me be careful and attentive as I am learning about this new situation.

How do I want to think about the physical reaction from now on?

It doesn't help to obsess about it because it just makes me more nervous. There's nothing wrong with me—I'm not sick or disgusting; I'm just excited. I try to remind myself that the other person could be nervous and excited too, and the noises will go away eventually. If they care so much about my stomach growling they probably aren't that nice anyway.

Example 2

A strong physical sensation with an emotion:

Every time I go into the dining hall my stomach feels really weird and bad—sometimes I feel nauseous, and sometimes I have pains in my stomach. I have pains after I eat, too.

How does this physical sensation feel dysfunctional?

I'm supposed to be eating! So feeling sick is totally counterproductive. Also it makes me feel like there might be something wrong with the food, the food could be bad for me, maybe it will make me sick, or something else that is bad will happen if I try to eat it.

How could this physical sensation actually be a normal and natural part of an emotion?

It is normal to have weird feelings in your stomach when you are anxious. That's again the muscle tension and the blood leaving the digestive system.

Is there anything that could even be functional about having that emotion?

I get anxious about food because I am afraid it is going to make me fat, and then it is normal for my stomach to have that reaction. If someone was trying to feed me something that really was going to hurt me, it would be good to be anxious and be able to run away. Though that isn't a very likely scenario outside of Game of Thrones or a detective novel.

How do I want to think about the physical reaction from now on?

I want to remember that my stomach hurting is my anxiety misfiring because I have been treating food like it is dangerous. It is not a signal that I am sick or that the food is going to be bad for me. It should go away over time if I lean into it.

Your turn

Now it's your turn to apply your own experiences. Can you think of two different examples and complete the exercise? Use the examples above to help you.

Your first example

A strong physical sensation with an emotion:

_____

_____

How does this physical sensation feel dysfunctional?

_____

_____

_____

_____

How could this physical sensation actually be a normal and natural part of an emotional reaction?

_____

_____

_____

_____

Is there anything that could even be functional about having that emotion?

_____

_____

_____

_____

How do I want to think about the physical reaction from now on?

_____

_____

_____

_____

Your second example

A strong physical sensation with an emotion:

_____

_____

How does this physical sensation feel dysfunctional?

_____

_____

How could this physical sensation actually be a normal and natural part of an emotional reaction?

_____

_____

_____

Is there anything that could even be functional about having that emotion?

_____

_____

_____

_____

How do I want to think about the physical reaction from now on?

_____

_____

_____

_____

The Three Parts of Emotions (3-Component Model)

GOALS

- Understand and describe the three components of emotions:
  - Thoughts
  - Physical sensations
  - Behaviors and urges

HOMEWORK REVIEW

- Fill out Form 3.1: Eating, Depression, and Anxiety (EDA).
- Plot scores on Form 3.2: EDA Graph.
- Fill out Form 4.1: Regular Eating Food Log.
- Read and complete Worksheet 6.1: Function of Physical Sensations Homework.
- Read Chapter 7 and preview the exercises.

Our goal for today is to understand the different parts of an emotion. This is the backbone of the work you will do to identify your emotions and get ready to change how you approach and experience them.

What makes up an emotion?

We have discussed how emotions can be functional or adaptive. As shown in Figure 7.1, every emotional experience can actually be broken down into three main parts—what we are thinking, what is happening in our body, and what we are doing.

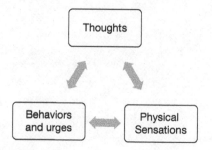

Figure 7.1:
The Three Parts of an Emotion

The three components of emotional experiences

1. Cognitive (what you think)

These are the thoughts often triggered by or linked with emotional states. For example, someone who is feeling sadness may have thoughts about a situation being hopeless, or being inadequate, such as, "I am screwing up again."

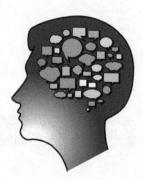

2. Physical (how your body feels)

These are the physical responses attached to emotional states, or the way your body physically demonstrates emotions. For example, fear may include a racing heart, a tensing of the muscles, or shortness of breath. Anxiety may be shown in your sweaty palms or a tightness or pain in the stomach or chest. Sadness may be accompanied by a sensation of heaviness in the limbs.

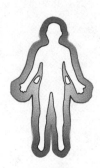

3. Behavioral (what you do, actions or urges)

These are actions a person does *or has the urge to do* as a response to the emotional state. Often, someone will respond to a feeling without thinking about it. These experiences are what we call "emotion-driven behaviors" or EDBs. You don't want to think; you just want to act quickly. EDBs may be present in emotional experiences that do not feel useful or adaptive. For example, someone who is depressed may stay in bed all day and might not eat anything because it is hard to face dealing with the day. Someone who is anxious in social settings may avoid eye contact, or avoid eating, or even leave the situation entirely.

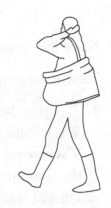

The 3-Component Model exercise

To get good at identifying the three parts of an emotional experience, we use something called the 3-Component Model. Emotions are complex, and we have to practice identifying the three parts—thoughts, physical sensations, and behaviors. These parts also interact with one another, and in the 3-Component Model we put two-way arrows from each part to the other parts to show how they all affect one another.

Let's think about how your eating symptoms fit into this model. Restricting, eating, and compensating are *behaviors*. Criticism of your body or your eating and specific fears about your body or eating are *thoughts*. So your eating disorder has a behavioral component, and it also has a cognitive component—that is, what you are thinking, about food, your body, your emotions, yourself, the situation, and so on. And there is also a physical component: Both before and after any behavior, there are physical sensations like "hunger" or "pain" that can be associated with eating, and there are physical sensations that go along with the emotional component of eating disorders such as anxiety, sadness, shame, or disgust.

Think of the last time you experienced a major symptom of your eating disorder, and diagram it on In-Session Exercise 7.1: The 3-Component Model.

In-Session Exercise 7.1
The 3-Component Model

Name the situation here: _____

Then in the corresponding circles below, write your answers to the following questions:

1. <u>Thoughts</u>: What thoughts were you having at that time? What was your brain telling you? Was it telling you anything about yourself? Was it making any predictions about the future? Was it saying something about the emotion itself? Have you been in similar situations? What thoughts came up in that situation?

2. <u>Physical Sensations</u>: What are the physical sensations associated with that emotion? Think about your stomach, head, chest, muscles . . . Think about heaviness, tightness, pain, numbness, tingling . . . What were you feeling in your body?

3. <u>Behaviors/Urges</u>: In this case, what did you do? What did you do immediately, in the situation? Did you do anything to reduce your discomfort? What *didn't* you do? Did you have any other urges that you didn't act on? What might you have done or felt like doing in other, similar situations?

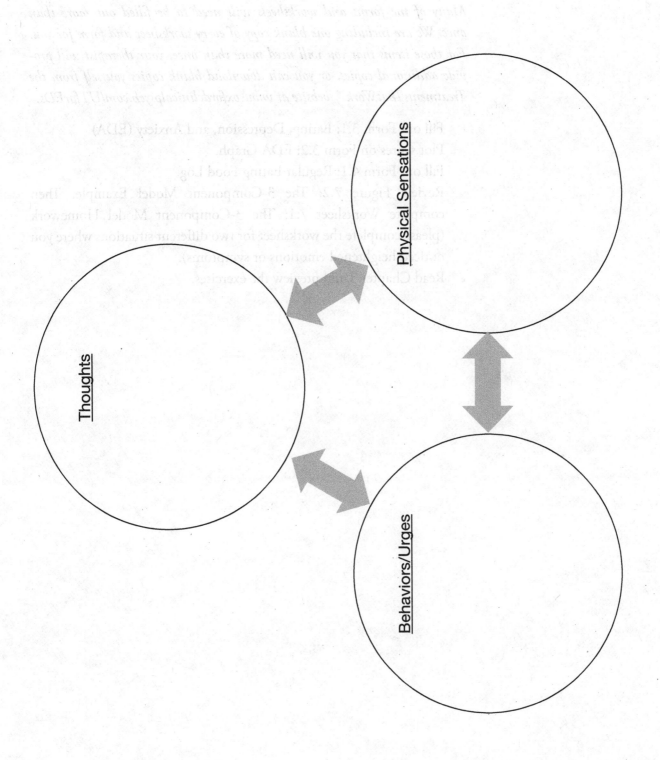

Many of the forms and worksheets will need to be filled out more than once. We are including one blank copy of every worksheet and form for you. For those items that you will need more than once, your therapist will provide additional copies, or you can download blank copies yourself from the Treatments That Work™ website at www.oxfordclinicalpsych.com/UTforEDs.

- Fill out Form 3.1: Eating, Depression, and Anxiety (EDA).
- Plot scores on Form 3.2: EDA Graph.
- Fill out Form 4.1: Regular Eating Food Log.
- Review Figure 7.2: The 3-Component Model Example. Then complete Worksheet 7.1: The 3-Component Model Homework (please complete the worksheet for two different situations where you noticed heightened emotions or symptoms).
- Read Chapter 8 and preview the exercises.

Names of emotions:

Anxiety, fear, anger

Situation:

Lunch

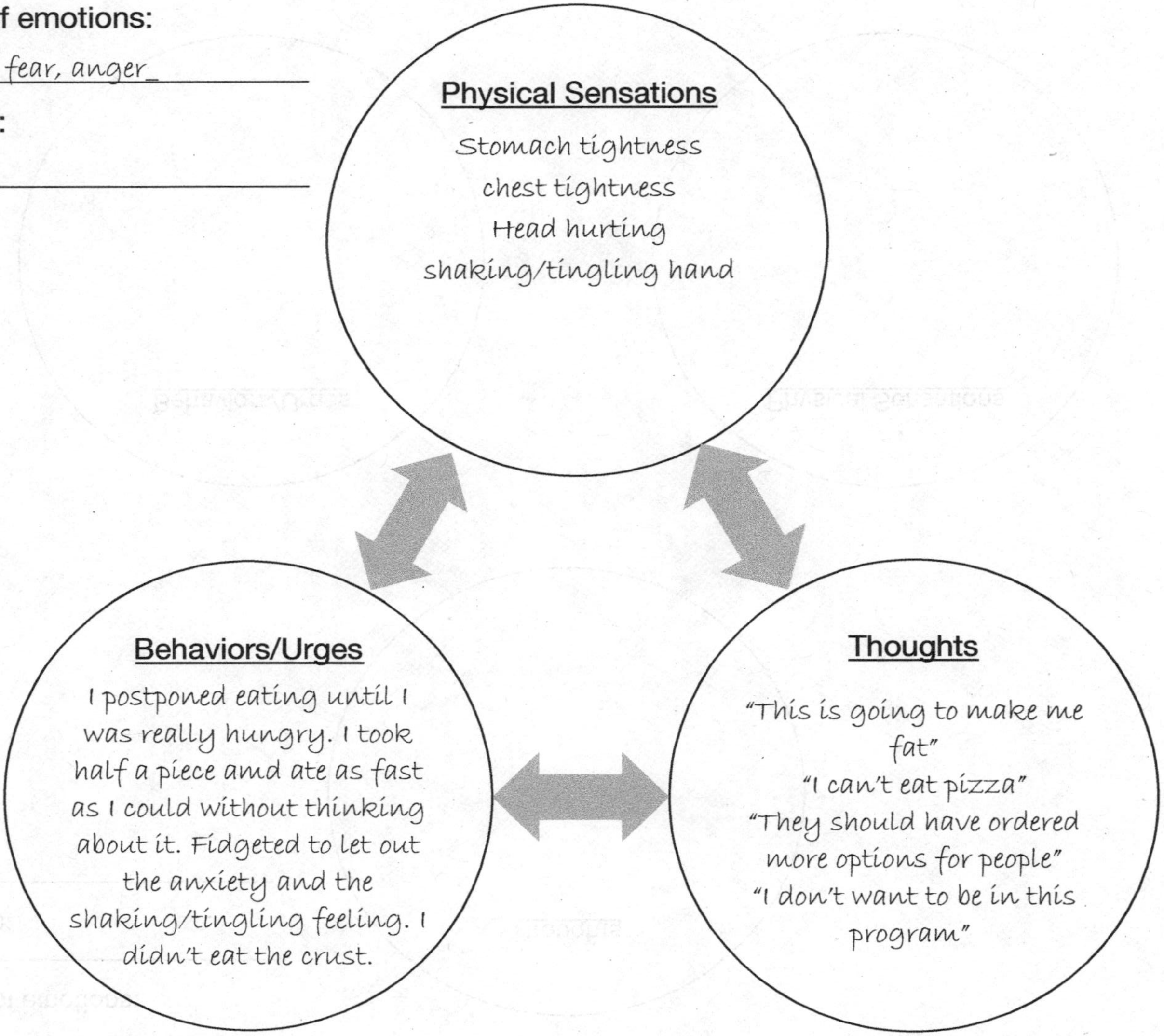

Physical Sensations

Stomach tightness
chest tightness
Head hurting
shaking/tingling hand

Thoughts

"This is going to make me
fat"
"I can't eat pizza"
"They should have ordered
more options for people"
"I don't want to be in this
program"

Behaviors/Urges

I postponed eating until I
was really hungry. I took
half a piece and ate as fast
as I could without thinking
about it. Fidgeted to let out
the anxiety and the
shaking/tingling feeling. I
didn't eat the crust.

Figure 7.2:

The 3-Component Model Example

Worksheet 7.1
The 3-Component Model Homework

Names of emotions:

_____

Situation: _____

Thoughts

Physical Sensations

Behaviors/Urges

Names of emotions: _____

Situation: _____

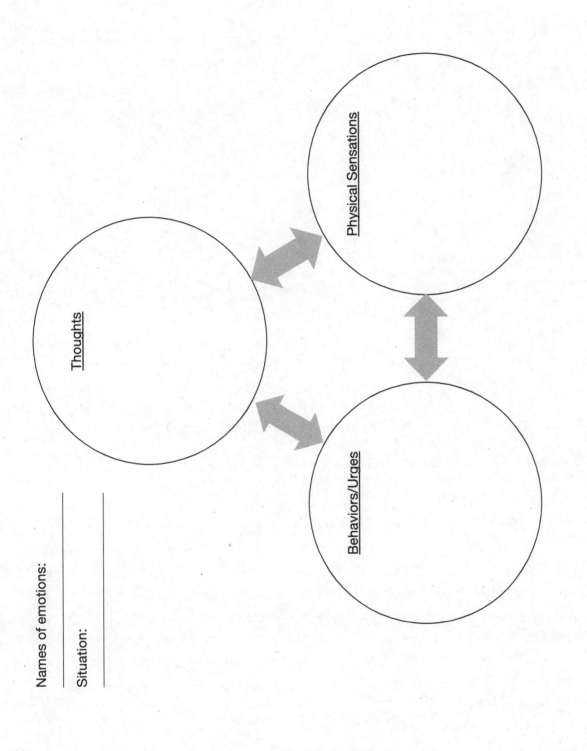

Thoughts

Physical Sensations

Behaviors/Urges

CHAPTER 8 — Tracking Emotions over Time (the "ARC")

- Learn the steps that unfold over time in emotions:
  - Antecedent (A)
  - Response (R)
  - Consequence (C)
- Look for patterns in your emotional triggers.
- Explore short- and long-term consequences of your emotional responses.

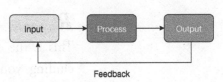

- Fill out Form 3.1: Eating, Depression, and Anxiety (EDA).
- Plot scores on Form 3.2: EDA Graph.
- Fill out Form 4.1: Regular Eating Food Log.
- Review Figure 7.2: The 3-Component Model Example. Then complete Worksheet 7.1: The 3-Component Model Homework (please complete the worksheet for two different situations where you noticed heightened emotions or symptoms).
- Read Chapter 8 and preview the exercises.

Our main goal for today is to explore and learn how emotional experiences unfold. This allows us to learn from our emotional experiences and how these experiences can influence our later behaviors and emotions. The ARC of emotions is meant to introduce you to the process of monitoring experiences. This allows for a better understanding of these experiences, enabling you to respond more flexibly. Every emotional experience we have is triggered by some event or situation, which causes us to react and respond, and these responses have consequences.

*A*ntecedent

This means what happened *before*. Think of all the situational factors, the triggers that happened immediately before, and even earlier, that created the context and set you up for the emotional experience.

*R*esponse

This is the emotional *reaction* or *response* to all of the antecedents, including your thoughts, physical sensations, and behaviors/urges. The R includes all three components that we talked about before, the three components that we put in the circles in Chapter 7.

*C*onsequences

These are all the results, everything—good and bad—that follows from your responses. Maybe you learned that was a useful reaction in some way. Maybe you didn't. Maybe you missed out on learning something you might have learned if you had taken a different action. We don't specifically mean negative consequences, or "punishment," but just all the outcomes—negative and positive—and particularly what you may have learned about your emotions as a result.

Take a look at Figure 8.1: The ARC of Emotional Experiences (Sample), and familiarize yourself with the layout.

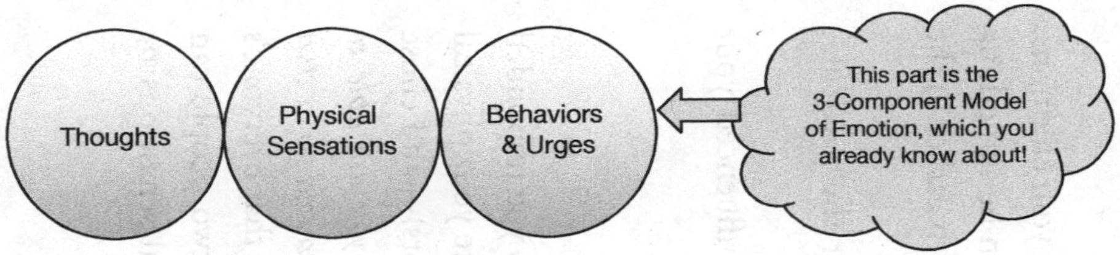

Figure 8.1:

The ARC of Emotional Experiences (Sample)

This part is the 3-Component Model of Emotion, which you already know about!

Thoughts — Physical Sensations — Behaviors & Urges

Date/Time	Antecedents (situation & triggers)	Responses			Consequences What happened next? What did you learn?
		Thoughts	Physical Sensations	Behaviors & Urges	
EMOTIONAL EVENT:	Immediate: Earlier:				Short-term: Long-term:
EMOTIONAL EVENT:	Immediate: Earlier:				Short-term: Long-term:

Here are a few important things to keep in mind at this stage:

☞ It is not important yet to record specific aspects of your experiences, such as strategies you might be using to manage your experiences, or avoid your emotions, or what you plan on doing next time.

☞ Your goal is to simply monitor your emotional experiences and to become more aware of the whole context in which these experiences occur.

☞ It is important to know that our emotional reactions are typically very automatic and we are not always fully aware of each part.

Workshop-style group ARC

Let's use a meal as an example to explain how the ARC works and to fill out Figure 8.1. Take a moment to clearly think about a recent meal. Instead of focusing on the food itself, we want you to focus on the emotional experience.

What is the A of your situation?

▪ As you begin to identify events or situations that trigger your emotions, it is also important to recognize that these triggers can be something that has just happened, something that happened much earlier in the day, or even something that happened last week.

▪ Can you think of other factors that set the stage for the particular reaction you had?

▪ How would a different type of day or week have influenced your reaction?

Next, let's do the R of your situation.

▪ Go through the 3-Components Model to describe how you responded to the situation. What were your thoughts? What were your physical sensations? What were the actions you took (behaviors)—and chose *not* to take—and what were the urges you felt? *If you are able to identify the actual emotion that you're describing, go ahead and write that next to the word "Responses."* It is important to notice that everyone's personal reaction is unique. In the same situation, two people can react differently, based on the thoughts and physical sensations or behaviors/urges they have.

We humans are designed to learn from experiences. The only way for us to know what is good and what is bad is through our experiences, and our emotions help to guide us in making this distinction. If we want to ensure our survival, we should move toward things that are good for us and away from things that are bad. Moving toward things that are good for us may also help us in other valuable ways—for example, feeling settled, being honest, feeling proud, being authentic, and feeling valued. *More often than not, it is our emotions that are telling us what is good or bad.*

As we have talked about before, this serves an adaptive purpose in nature. For example, if a rabbit in the forest comes across a fox lurking in the bushes near a watering hole, the intense emotion of fear that the rabbit experiences helps the rabbit to learn that it should stay away from this potentially life-threatening situation in the future. The rabbit learns very quickly from this experience of fear in order to ensure its survival. This type of learning takes place in nature all the time and just goes to show that even if we don't necessarily like fear, fear definitely has its place and is a very helpful emotion.

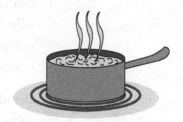

This type of learning is something people share and has been passed down through evolution. As humans, we too are designed to learn quickly from our experiences. For example, if you are cooking on a stove and accidentally grab a pot handle that is very hot, you experience pain and immediately pull your hand away. When you reach for a pot handle the next time, you may stop yourself and grab a potholder instead in order to avoid the painful experience of being burned again. What's more, we are also designed to quickly apply what we have learned to other similar situations. For example, you not only stop yourself from grabbing the handle of the pot that burned you before, but you also hesitate before grabbing other handles on other stoves or hot surfaces. We are hard-wired to learn this way.

So, what does this have to do with your symptoms? We quickly learn and alter our behavior in response to unpleasant emotional experiences. When we have unpleasant emotional experiences, we may learn to *escape* or *avoid.*

A lot of this learning is adaptive, but it is not always so. What about if we *escaped from fear* by dropping the food and running away every time we feel fear of gaining weight? Or how about avoiding the unpleasant emotion of embarrassment by avoiding all social gatherings? Sometimes we interpret our emotions as guiding us away from a threatening situation that might not even be there, and our responses in turn become unhelpful (maladaptive) instead of helpful (adaptive).

Part of the aim of this program is to help you make the distinction between real threats and *perceived* threats, so you can be more flexible about how to respond to your emotions.

Emotion-driven behaviors, or EDBs, in response to negative emotions make sense because they *relieve the emotion and help us to avoid feeling worse*. For example, we might use eating disorder symptoms to relieve anxiety; or quickly exit a crowded area when feeling panicky; or stay in bed all day when feeling down. Over time, however, we learn to do this same EDB repertoire over and over again in an attempt to relieve the emotion and the possibility of feeling worse. The problem is that repeatedly doing these EDBs can result in a vicious cycle where EDBs become automatic and counterproductive and don't relate to the true context in which our behavior is occurring.

Because EDBs relieve uncomfortable emotions in the short term, we may think they are useful for us, even though they also may be interfering with our ability to live our lives.

These learned strategies for coping with intense emotions, such as avoiding situations that trigger emotions, have important effects on the C (consequences) phase of the ARC model. By avoiding these strong and intense feelings, we never have the chance to find out what these feelings might really be telling us, or to see that *these feelings will pass*. And by avoiding intense emotions, we may actually be depriving ourselves of important, valued aspects of our lives.

Going back to the meal example, let's think more about the C: What were the consequences of your different responses? There is a short-term consequence that is different from the long-term consequence. With EDBs, sometimes the short-term consequence is to feel better, or to stop feeling distressed, whereas the long-term consequences are more problematic. On the other hand, deciding to be uncomfortable in the short term might feel like a terrible idea, but there might be a long-term payoff that's really good for you. See Figure 8.2: An Example of the Emotion–Behavior–Consequences Cycle.

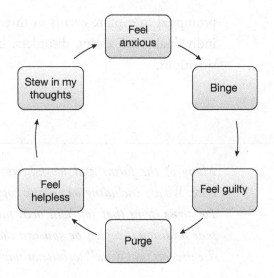

Figure 8.2:

An Example of the Emotion–Behavior–Consequences Cycle

Explanation of this session's homework

The homework is to do your own ARC of emotions. You can choose any emotional experience that is current for you. We really want you to focus on this experience vividly, so it's best if it's fresh in your mind. Do your ARC just like we did in session together using Form 8.1.

Try to do at least one ARC every day. Remember, the point of the ARC is not to reduce your emotion but rather to help you track it and understand how the emotion unfolds. This is a skill worth developing, and it requires practice!

You also need to complete Worksheet 8.1: Following Your Thoughts. This is an important exercise for your next ARC session and will really help you become aware of how many different types of thoughts might be happening simultaneously in an emotional experience. To complete Worksheet 8.1, you can choose any one of the experiences that you completed the ARC for, and follow the prompts to identify as many thoughts as possible. We will be diving into this material in the next session.

Next you will need to complete Worksheet 8.2: Focusing on Your Behaviors. This exercise will increase your awareness of your behaviors and help you start identifying what the function of those behaviors might be. Spoiler alert: These behaviors probably help you escape or avoid uncomfortable emotions. What's nice about this exercise is that you are prompted to explore events in three categories that are quite relevant to individuals with eating disorders: body image, food, and interpersonal situations.

Homework

Many of the forms and worksheets will need to be filled out more than once. We are including one blank copy of every worksheet and form for you. For those items that you will need more than once, your therapist will provide additional copies, or you can download blank copies yourself from the TreatmentsThatWork™ website at www.oxfordclinicalpsych.com/UTforEDs.

- Fill out Form 3.1: Eating, Depression, and Anxiety (EDA).
- Plot scores on Form 3.2: EDA Graph.
- Fill out Form 4.1: Regular Eating Food Log.
- Complete the full Form 8.1: The ARC of Emotional Experiences for:
  - A body image event
  - A food/eating event
  - An event related to another emotional goal (fill in goal here):

  _____

  _____

- Complete Worksheet 8.1: Following Your Thoughts and Worksheet 8.2: Focusing on Your Behaviors.
- Read Chapter 9 and preview the exercises.

Form 8.1

The ARC of Emotional Experiences

Date/ Time	Antecedents (situation & triggers)	Responses			Consequences (what happened next?)
		Thoughts	Physical Sensations	Behaviors & Urges	
EMOTIONAL EVENT:	Immediate:				Short-term:
	Earlier:				Long-term:
EMOTIONAL EVENT:	Immediate:				Short-term:
	Earlier:				Long-term:

Worksheet 8.1
Following Your Thoughts

The situation: _____

1. What were your foremost thoughts about the situation?

_____

_____

2. What thoughts did you have about anyone else who was involved?

_____

_____

3. What thoughts did you have about the emotion itself?

_____

_____

4. What thoughts did you have specifically about the physical sensations?

_____

_____

5. What thoughts did you have about your ability to handle the emotion?

_____

_____

6. What thoughts did you have that were judgments of the emotion?

_____

_____

7. What thoughts did you have about yourself as a person?

_____

_____

8. What thoughts did you have about similar situations that happened in the past?

_____

_____

9. What thoughts did you have that were predictions about the future?

_____

_____

10. Did you have thoughts about what you should do?

_____

_____

Worksheet 8.2
Focusing on Your Behaviors

You are going to record events in three categories: emotions about body image, food, and inter-personal events. List as many behaviors as you can. A "behavior" can be to do nothing, as well as to do something—like "stay in the room" or "sit with it" rather than leaving or reacting in another way. Then try to rate that behavior as to how *avoidant* it was on a scale from 0 to 8, where *0 = not at all avoidant*, fully leaning-in, doing nothing except allowing for the experience of emotion, or doing something that represents going "toward" emotion; and *8 = highly avoidant*, with a highly emotionally driven and urgent effort to escape from the emotion and situation. The goal is to help raise your awareness of your behaviors, so don't worry too much about whether you get the rating "exactly right."

0	1	2	3	4	5	6	7	8
Not avoidant			Compromise			Highly escapist/avoidant		

Emotional Events	Actual Behaviors You Used	Escape/Avoidance Rating
Body Image Emotional Event		
Food-Related Emotional Event		
_____-Related Emotional Event		

Mindful Emotion Awareness

- Understand the concepts involved in mindfulness:
  - Awareness of two types of emotion, primary and secondary
  - Awareness that is present-focused, not focused on the past or future
  - Awareness that is accepting of emotion rather than judgmental

- Fill out Form 3.1: Eating, Depression, and Anxiety (EDA).
- Plot scores on Form 3.2: EDA Graph.
- Fill out Form 4.1: Regular Eating Food Log.
- Complete the full Form 8.1: The ARC of Emotional Experiences for:
  - A body image event
  - A food/eating event
  - An event related to another emotional goal (fill in goal here):

  _____

- Complete Worksheet 8.1: Following Your Thoughts and Worksheet 8.2: Focusing on Your Behaviors.
- Read Chapter 9 and preview the exercises.

Mindfulness is a state of being fully aware. We are focusing our awareness and attention on the present moment while acknowledging and accepting our emotion of the moment, and our thoughts, behaviors/urges, and bodily sensations. Figure 9.1: What Is Mindfulness? outlines the components of mindfulness.

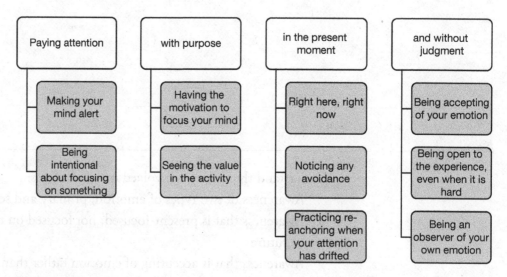

Figure 9.1:

What Is Mindfulness?

Today, we will focus on the issue of judgment, including *primary and secondary emotions*.

Awareness of primary and secondary emotions

As illustrated in Figure 9.2: Diagram of a Primary Emotion, within every emotional experience there is an initial emotion triggered by some event or thought, which is then followed by a reaction to this emotion.

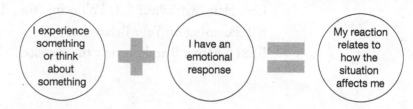

Figure 9.2:

Diagram of a Primary Emotion

Often this initial emotion, called a *primary emotion*, is not in and of itself a problem, such as a sudden surge of fear in response to an unexpected noise, or feeling sad when you get some bad news. There are so many ways that we adaptively respond to or demonstrate our primary emotions through the three components of thoughts, behaviors, and physiological sensations.

Primary emotions are the "first" emotional response/reaction to a situation or memory, and these reactions are often *functional* and *directly related* to the cues in the situation/thought.

But there can be another layer to this. We call this *a secondary emotion.* Secondary emotions are a response to the primary emotional response. Secondary emotions are often unhelpful, as illustrated in Figure 9.3: Diagram of a Secondary Emotion.

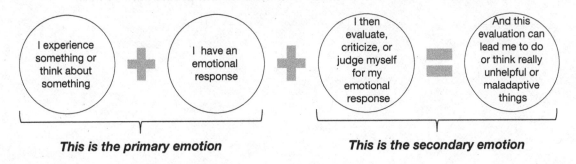

Figure 9.3:

Diagram of a Secondary Emotion

Sometimes we *criticize* ourselves or the emotion itself. Sometimes we are harsh with ourselves about how we reacted to a primary emotion, or we think the emotion is unbearable, and then things can become problematic. Let's take an example of sadness. You're having a really hard time at the moment and feel very sad, so you begin to cry. That sounds like a primary emotion, which can exist on its own without any negative consequences. However, if you criticize yourself for crying, saying, "I'm being silly; this shouldn't make me cry; I need to pull myself together," you might feel ashamed of crying or angry with yourself for being weak. The shame and anger are the *secondary emotions*, and these feelings might result in using an avoidant, unhelpful behavior to make yourself stop feeling sadness. *Secondary emotions are the ways we react to primary emotions we don't want to feel.*

Secondary reactions to emotions are often evaluative or judgmental, such as when we believe that anxiety is a sign that we can't cope with the current situation, that sadness is a sign we are a failure or that the situation is hopeless, or that physical fullness is a sign that we will become dangerously overweight. These responses often lead to problematic behaviors/urges. Problematic avoidance strategies and emotion-driven behaviors (EDBs) are part of the secondary emotion. Our goal is to stick with the primary emotion, for now.

In summary, *secondary emotions*:

- Are not based on the present moment,
- Can be judgmental reactions to the primary emotional response,
- May prevent us from taking in corrective information in a situation that is useful, and
- May drive our use of avoidance and problematic EDBs.

In-Session Exercise 9.1
Awareness of Primary Emotions and Secondary Emotions

There are six emotional states listed below; these are situations that many of us may identify with. The main point of this activity is to explore different ways to respond to emotional states, including our usual secondary (judgmental) reactions, and also helpful and adaptive ways:

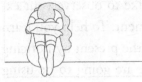

- ◾ I'm having a really hard time at the moment and *I feel very sad*, so I:
  - ◾ Usual secondary reactions?_____
  - ◾ Adaptive reactions?_____

- ◾ I'm going to see my weight today and *I'm so afraid* of what the number will be, so I:
  - ◾ Usual secondary reactions?_____
  - ◾ Adaptive reactions?_____

- ◾ *I was really angry* at my friend, so I:
  - ◾ Usual secondary reactions?_____
  - ◾ Adaptive reactions?_____

- ◾ Now *I feel so guilty* about how I treated my friend, so I:
  - ◾ Usual secondary reactions?_____
  - ◾ Adaptive reactions?_____

- ◾ Something really wonderful just happened to me and *I'm overjoyed*, so I:
  - ◾ Usual secondary reactions?_____
  - ◾ Adaptive reactions?_____

- ◾ My plans were canceled last minute, *and I feel lonely*, so I:
  - ◾ Usual secondary reactions?_____
  - ◾ Adaptive reactions?_____

- ◾ I'm chilling out at home alone, *feeling quite bored*, so I:
  - ◾ Usual secondary reactions?_____
  - ◾ Adaptive reactions?_____

In-Session Exercise 9.2
Guided Mindfulness

> It's not a matter of letting go – you would if you could. Instead of "Let it go," we should probably say "Let it be."
> – Jon Kabat–Zinn

Now that you have fully explored possible secondary reactions, we want you to start practicing paying close attention to your experience.

It is important to get used to what it feels like to observe your experience as it is occurring in the present moment. To help you learn this skill, let's practice anchoring yourself to the present by noticing at least one thing going on around you. We are going to be using Worksheet 9.1: Nonjudgmental Present-Focused Emotion Awareness (located later in this chapter) for homework.

First, let's focus on physical sensations. Close your eyes and for a moment now, turn your attention to yourself in the room. Picture the room—imagine what the room looks like, what is in the room, where the furniture is laid out. Now picture yourself sitting inside the room and exactly where you are. Notice how it feels to be sitting in the chair. Begin to observe how your body feels and any sensations that are there. Notice any physical reactions you are having. Pause for a moment, and just allow yourself to observe your physical sensations. What physical sensations did you notice? Jot these things down on Worksheet 9.2.

Next, let's focus on the present moment. To anchor yourself in the present, one very useful cue is the breath. Pairing a deep breath with a shift in attention onto something tangible occurring in the present moment (such as listening to the sounds around you) can condition the breath to serve as a powerful cue to remind you to focus on the present moment. However, breath here is not intended to be a distraction or relaxation technique. Rather, breath here serves as a reminder to focus on what is going on at this moment.

Now, let's try using breath as a way to anchor ourselves. Slowly bring your attention to your own breathing. Notice yourself breathing in and breathing out. Focus on your breathing as it is happening right now, in this moment, using your breath to help anchor yourself to the present moment. Focus on the sensation of your breath entering your body, then leaving your body. Your breath is always with you, and your breathing is always happening in the here and now. Use your breath to remind you to pay attention and observe what is happening right now. Pause for a moment, and just allow yourself to notice your breath. What did you notice?

In-Session Exercise 9.3
Focusing on Nonjudgmental Emotion Awareness

The goal of this exercise is not to think about the meaning of what you notice, nor is it to try to understand your reaction to it. The goal is to let go of judgments about your experience and to just practice being an observer of your own experience or reactions. In this sense, there is no "right" or "wrong" way, just getting more used to observing how your thoughts, physical sensations, and behaviors unfold and influence each other. Remember, you are practicing becoming a curious observer of your experience, rather than approaching your experience as a judge and jury like you might be used to doing. This is a new perspective, and it takes time to get comfortable with it.

Let's try some more exercises together, using Worksheet 9.1: Nonjudgmental Present-Focused Emotion Awareness to continue taking notes.

As you stay focused on your breath, bring your attention inward toward your own thoughts. Notice how your thoughts are constantly changing. Sometimes you think one way, sometimes you think another. Some thoughts just pass by, others may distract you, and some of them may be hard to let go of. Simply notice what you're thinking. If you notice yourself getting caught up in or carried away by a thought, just acknowledge it, without judgment, and gently try to bring your attention back to observing your thoughts as they occur. Allow yourself to watch your thoughts for a few moments—and as you do, notice how they come and go.

What did you notice?

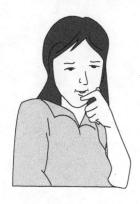

As you take note of these thoughts, start to shift and explore how you're feeling. Emotions, just like thoughts, are constantly changing. Sometimes you feel love and sometimes hatred, sometimes calm and then tense, joyful and then sorrowful, happy and then sad. Sometimes emotions come in waves, sometimes they linger; sometimes they are brought on by certain thoughts, other times they seem to come out of nowhere. Simply acknowledge how you're feeling in this very moment. Allow yourself to observe your emotions, without judgment. Notice how they ebb and flow. Pause for a moment, and just allow yourself to observe your emotions.

What did you notice?

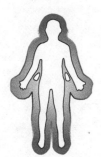

Continuing to use your breath to anchor you, begin to take note of your entire experience— how your body feels, what you are thinking, what emotions you are experiencing. If you notice that you are trying to change your experience in some way, take note of that, and gently guide yourself back to your experience. Notice whatever you're experiencing in this very moment.

What did you notice?

 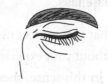

Using your breath to anchor you, allow your awareness to shift so you can take in what's going on around you. Notice the temperature of the room. Notice any sounds occurring outside the room. Notice any sounds occurring inside the room.

What did you notice?

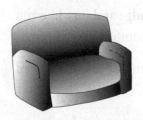

And, when you are ready, start to bring yourself back into the room. Picture yourself sitting in this room, picture the way the room looks, how it is laid out. When you are ready, come back into the room and open your eyes.

As you can see by this example, doing this exercise the first time around may feel a little strange, or you may feel like you are not doing it right. Remember that the goal of this exercise is not to do it perfectly; rather, the goal is to begin to learn how to observe and be aware of your own experience, to understand how the whole process unfolds for you. This will help you to begin to see where your emotional experiences might be changing from something adaptive and helpful to something maladaptive and unhelpful.

Homework

Many of the forms and worksheets will need to be filled out more than once. We are including one blank copy of every worksheet and form for you. For those items that you will need more than once, your therapist will provide additional copies, or you can download blank copies yourself from the TreatmentsThatWork™ website at www.oxfordclinicalpsych.com/UTforEDs.

- Fill out Form 3.1: Eating, Depression, and Anxiety (EDA).
- Plot scores on Form 3.2: EDA Graph.
- Fill out Form 4.1: Regular Eating Food Log.
- Complete Form 8.1: The ARC of Emotional Experiences.
- You are going to practice nonjudgmental, present-focused awareness this week, daily, for homework. Choose one situation, per day, for the next week where you can practice present-focused awareness. It can be just sitting quietly, doing a mindful walk (as described in Worksheet 9.3: Present-Focused Awareness Exercise I—Mindful Walking), listening to a song, washing the dishes, or any other 5-minute period of time during the day. Use Worksheet 9.1: Nonjudgmental Present-Focused Emotion Awareness, and record one entry per night.
- You are going to be generating examples of secondary emotions and exploring the effect of these reactions. Please review Figure 9.4: Primary and Secondary Emotions Worksheet and Box 9.1 on your own to help you better understand this concept, and then complete Worksheet 9.2. Your therapist will guide you through the two practice examples on the figures and explain the worksheet instructions carefully.
- Do a daily mindfulness practice: Sit and breathe, or do a mindful walk, and then complete Worksheet 9.1.
- Read Chapter 10 and preview the exercises.

Worksheet 9.1
Nonjudgmental Present-Focused Emotion Awareness

You can choose to sit and breathe for this exercise, or try the mindful walk described in Worksheet 9.3. Anchor yourself to the present by anchoring yourself to your breath. Then you can be creative about what you want to intentionally focus on. This can be a sound you hear, something you see, or something you can physically feel (like your chair, or a breeze, or a sound). The two goals are to try to be here and now (not in the future or past) and to notice when you are judging and redirect to nonjudgmental awareness. When you are finished, fill out the entry in the worksheet.

	Describing what you noticed: What physical sensations (such as hearing, smelling, seeing, and feeling) did you notice? Did any emotions arise for you? What else did you notice?	How much did you stay in the present? 0–10 (0 = completely lost in past or future; 10 = totally in the here and now)	How much did you accept your experiences? 0–10 (0 = all judging; 10 = totally accepting)
In Session			
Day 1			
Day 2			
Day 3			
Day 4			
Day 5			
Day 6			

What is a Primary Emotion?	What is a Secondary Emotion?
It is the core emotion or the "true" emotion that matches the situation or memory	Is the "emotion about the emotion"
Some people call it the "first" emotional reaction to the situation or memory	In other words, it is your reaction to your primary emotion
It is often adaptive and functional	It is often judgmental, self-critical, or evaluative
It is directly related to the situation or memory	It is not typically based on the present moment
It leads to adaptive behaviors (i.e., not to avoidance or EDBs)	It often leads to the use of avoidance and EDBs

Examples

Sadness → Shame/anger/blaming

"Mom was supposed to visit, but then she cancelled last minute. I was really looking forward to this, and now this is so disappointing and upsetting. I can't stop the tears from streaming down my cheeks."

"Typical; I can't hold it together. I just cry for anything. People must think I'm such a loser for crying like this. Screw this; this is so stupid! This is my mom's fault! She is always so inconsiderate and flaky. I should have never asked her to come anyway. She always lets me down and makes me feel this way; she doesn't care about me."

Anxiety → Shame

"Eating this meal plan is so difficult for me, and anything that is not a 'safe food' makes me really uncomfortable and triggers my urges. I am so scared right now."

"I am so pathetic. Chicken and rice is so 'normal.' I can't believe I can't do this! Why can't I just eat like a normal person? My whole family can't understand why I can't do this."

Fear → Embarrassment/anger

(Someone enters the room abruptly and I gasp weirdly and startle due to the unexpected noise.) "OMG, that frightened the you-know-what out of me. OMG, my heart is beating out of my chest. I got such a huge fright."

"Ah geez, I made a really weird and silly noise... urg, how humiliating. Everyone is looking at me. You stupid idiot, why did you have to come in here so suddenly?! What's wrong with you? Who opens the doors so loudly and abruptly?!"

Figure 9.4:

Primary and Secondary Emotions Worksheet

Box 9.1
Primary and Secondary Emotions Homework Activity

You have focused on the concept of primary and secondary emotions. If you're still feeling a little unclear about what those are, don't forget to review Figure 9.4: Primary and Secondary Emotions Worksheet. If you still have questions, that's understandable!

For this homework activity, you are going to generate your own personal examples of secondary emotions and explore what the problems with these reactions are. It is important not to be hypothetical in this exercise; instead, "dig deep" and really search for the things that you know you experience. Instead of exploring primary responses (directly related to the situation and possibly therefore helpful), we will explore secondary responses (often judgmental, maladaptive, or unhelpful). The goal of this homework is to:

- Identify your secondary response/reaction for each emotional state, and then
- Think of some problems or consequences that are associated with each secondary reaction.

Here are two examples to help you:

Feeling angry: Let's say you feel really <u>angry</u> (primary) with your friend, but then you start feeling <u>guilty</u> (secondary) for being <u>angry</u> (primary) with your friend. You judge yourself for being angry, and fear your friend would be angry if she knew, so you decide to just act like everything is alright.

What is the secondary reaction in this situation?

<u>I judged my initial feelings of anger even though they were valid, and instead I guilted myself into feeling like I was being silly for being angry, like it was a bad idea to be angry.</u>

What are some of the problems with this reaction?

- <u>I anticipated a bad future outcome because I thought that expressing my true feelings would cause a problem in our friendship, and she could reject me.</u>
- <u>I miss out on seeing that she actually may apologize and things would get better.</u>

Feeling sad: Now take the example of <u>sadness</u> (primary) and <u>depression</u> (secondary). Let's say in response to waking up and feeling terrible and pretty sad (primary), you conclude that you are just a worthless person for being so depressed (secondary) and you better stay in bed all day.

What is the secondary reaction in this situation?

<u>I let my depression take over and spiral downwards. So instead of feeling sad and trying to accept that and live with that experience, it suddenly became a major problem, and I felt like a total failure who couldn't face the world for the day.</u>

What are some of the problems with this reaction?

- <u>The judgment I made just makes me feel worse, more depressed, more incompetent.</u>
- <u>By staying in bed I miss the chance to learn that I could function while sad, and that I'm more competent than I might think.</u>

Worksheet 9.2
Primary and Secondary Emotions Homework

Think of some recent situations in which you felt the primary emotional state that is listed for each example. How did you judge or evaluate this experience in some way, which resulted in a secondary emotional response? Also describe some of the problems with each secondary reaction:

Feeling sad (primary) _____

_____

What is the secondary reaction in this situation? _____

_____

_____

What are some of the problems with this reaction?

_____

_____

Feeling nervous (primary) _____

_____

What is the secondary reaction in this situation?

_____

_____

What are some of the problems with this reaction?

_____

_____

Feeling guilty (primary) _____

_____

What is the secondary reaction in this situation?

_____

_____

What are some of the problems with this reaction?

_____

_____

Feeling joyful (primary) _____

_____

What is the secondary reaction in this situation?

_____

_____

What are some of the problems with this reaction?

_____

_____

Feeling bored (primary) _____

_____

What is the secondary reaction in this situation?

_____

_____

What are some of the problems with this reaction?

_____

_____

Feeling angry (primary) _____

_____

What is the secondary reaction in this situation?

_____

_____

What are some of the problems with this reaction?

_____

_____

If you find it hard to sit and breathe as a mindfulness activity, you might try mindful walking.

Choose a short path	• Chose a strip of floor, about 5–10 paces long. You are going to use this strip to walk back and forth along during the 5 minutes of mindful walking.
Prepare your feet	• You can chose to have bare feet, or keep your socks or shoes on—whatever will help you to focus and stay present.
Stay silent	• It's ideal to stay silent and really focus all of your attention on the task.
Do the mindful walk	• Walk slowly and intentionally, focusing on the bottoms of your feet. Use the physical sensations in your feet as an anchor to the present moment. Notice any emotion that arises.
Practice anchoring into the present moment	• As you're walking practice doing your 3-point check, and tune into the emotion that arises for you in response to the activity.

- **I'm paying attention <u>on purpose</u>.**

  - Notice the physical sensations of walking, the shifting of the weight, the pressure on your feet, the temperature of the floor, how your muscles work together to make a step possible.
  - Notice your thoughts and keep refocusing on thinking about the activity. You may notice that you are distracted, you may notice a judgmental thought, you may notice yourself "thinking about thinking." Try not to judge; just do your best to refocus.
  - Notice your behaviors or urges and any particular emotions that you feel.

- **I'm paying attention <u>with purpose</u>.**

As you walk, try to focus your attention on one or more sensations that you would normally take for granted, such as your breath coming in and out of your body and the movement of your feet and legs or their contact with the ground or floor.

- **What do I do if my mind wanders?** That's OK; it's perfectly natural. When you notice your mind wandering, simply use the breath or the physical sensations of the feet to anchor into the activity once again.

- **How do I walk?** Try to find a walk that feels natural, and not something exaggerated or stylized that will end up distracting you. You can do whatever feels most comfortable and natural with your hands and arms.

GOALS

- Review the principles of the natural course of emotions.
- Learn how mood induction is intended to help promote new tolerance of emotion.
- Plan mood induction exercises.

HOMEWORK REVIEW

- Fill out Form 3.1: Eating, Depression, and Anxiety (EDA).
- Plot scores on Form 3.2: EDA Graph.
- Fill out Form 4.1: Regular Eating Food Log.
- Complete Form 8.1: The ARC of Emotional Experiences.
- You are going to practice nonjudgmental, present-focused awareness this week, daily, for homework. Choose one situation, per day, for the next week where you can practice present-focused awareness. It can be just sitting quietly, doing a mindful walk (as described in Worksheet 9.3: Present-Focused Awareness Exercise I—Mindful Walking), listening to a song, washing the dishes, or any other 5-minute period of time during the day. Use Worksheet 9.1: Nonjudgmental Present-Focused Emotion Awareness and record one entry per night.
- You are going to be generating examples of secondary emotions and exploring the effect of these reactions. Please review Figure 9.4 and

Box 9.1 on your own to help you better understand this concept, and then complete Worksheet 9.2. Your therapist will guide you through the two practice examples on the figures and explain the worksheet instructions carefully.

- Do a daily mindfulness practice: Sit and breathe, or do a mindful walk, and then complete Worksheet 9.1.
- Read Chapter 10 and preview the exercises.

Mood induction: cultivating emotion awareness

By now you have a pretty good idea about the three components of emotion and also how emotional experiences unfold over time. Hopefully you are also starting to notice that some of the behaviors that you engage in when you experience strong emotions are intended to make those emotions go away—either by avoiding them in the first place or by reducing them or escaping them.

Consider the graph in Figure 10.1: The Natural Course of Emotion.

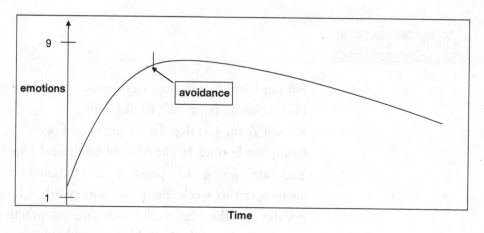

Figure 10.1:
The Natural Course of Emotion

On the x-axis (sideways) we have time going by (from left to right), and on the y-axis (up-and-down) we have the strength of the emotion (from 1 to 9). The general idea is that when something happens to provoke an emotion (point 1), that emotion will rise as time goes by. If we had to allow that emotion to rise, get to a peak, and then come down naturally, that would follow what we call the normal or natural course of emotion. However, sometimes we experience our emotions as unpleasant, and then we do things to make that unpleasant experience go away. When we do things to try to avoid our emotions, take the edge off, or stop them from occurring when they are at or near their most intense peak in a given situation, we add fuel to that emotion and will associate that situation in the future with these intense emotions.

Now we want to start stressing that one of the negative consequences of avoiding or escaping from emotion is that you never get to learn that if you have an uncomfortable emotion, and you don't judge it or try to escape from it, then the emotion is going to rise for a while and then come under control on its own. This may be hard to believe, but it hopefully will get easier over time.

So, you may be starting to notice that you *don't have to take these actions* for your emotions to come under control. Like we have said before, often the initial primary emotion isn't so overwhelming itself, and it is the reaction that we have to it that is more uncomfortable. A lot of us have the idea that the feeling *is just going to keep getting worse* or the thought that *you can't stand the*  *feeling*. Those are scary thoughts, and we have a secondary emotional response to them. These are the thoughts that lead to efforts to control or escape from the emotion. The truth is, if you experience an emotion as unpleasant, the quickest way to have that emotion diminish is to actually let it unfold! If you don't judge the emotion—rush to escape from it, suppress it, or make it go away—then it will come down by itself. Our bodies and our minds take care of this naturally.

However, there is a skill to develop when it comes to secondary emotions. The skill is to learn to not let those secondary reactions get in your way—to instead stick with the primary emotion—and to stop doing things that allow you to escape from the emotion or uncomfortable situations. If you can do that, and really let yourself experience your primary emotion, then you will start to develop a new tolerance of the emotions themselves.

The point of the mood induction exercises is to give you practice at allowing a primary emotion to occur naturally—to rise, peak, and fall again—and for you to notice that and also start noticing if you try to avoid certain emotions. This session has some specific themes: food, eating, and body image. This is because certain foods, eating, and our own bodies can elicit a powerful emotional response.

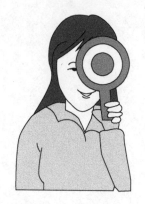

In-Session Exercise 10.1
Mood Induction Using Audio/Visual Media

Our in-session exercise is to try to feel some emotions deliberately by listening to some recordings of songs. We are going to start deliberately observing what we do when we actually have these more difficult emotions. We are going to practice doing general exercises in session so that we can then plan what to do that would be more specific to you and your emotions at home.

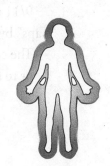

Please turn to Form 10.1: Mood Induction Recording at the end of this chapter. Notice what we are going to do, what boxes you are going to be filling in after the experiential part of the exercise is over. *The goal is to notice the thoughts, physical sensations, and behaviors/urges that come up during an emotional experience*.

Now, take a look back at Figure 9.4: Primary and Secondary Emotions Worksheet and review the concepts there. It's possible that you will try a mood induction exercise and not have a secondary emotion. Once these two forms make sense to you, you can put them aside.

Remember, the point of these exercises is for you to let an emotional experience happen, and to *notice what that experience is*, be it primary or secondary. The experience might be that you don't have very much of a reaction at all, and you will notice that. You might notice that you are afraid of the reaction and that you try pushing it away. The experience might be that you have a strong reaction, like feeling very tearful, angry, or guilty.

Of course, as in any session, you have choices about what you want to do with that emotion. The suggestion here is to try to have the emotion without judging it, to allow it to exist, to observe it, and to notice what happens with your thoughts, physical feelings, and behaviors. Try to remember that it is not dangerous to have emotions, but you may have been treating them as dangerous for a long time.

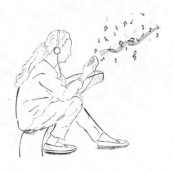

For this in-session exercise we have music that pretty reliably induces some emotions, of some kinds, in most people. There is no particular emotion that you should feel, and you may not feel that much. The goal is to see what you feel, let your emotion become as strong as you can without resisting it, notice if you have secondary emotions that take you away from the primary emotion, and discuss the experience afterward. It is a practice exercise for being able to plan this for yourself here and at home. We will do a few of them, so that hopefully one will resonate with you.

- Pharrell Williams singing "Happy"
    - The context of this song is that it comes from a moment in *Despicable Me 2* when the lead character has fallen in love.
- Whitney Houston singing "The Star-Spangled Banner"
    - The context of this recording is that Whitney Houston sang this version soon after the 9/11 terrorist attacks on the World Trade Center.
- "Taps" by the Army National Guard
    - The context of "Taps" is that it is a song played to say goodnight at the end of the day, or to say goodbye to a person who has died.

Explanation of this session's homework

Your job for homework is to do your own mood induction. Please feel free to repeat the exercise as many times as you like, each time monitoring any changes in your emotions. You should know what you are going to do before you leave today. Write down your idea, and brainstorm with the group leader if you need help accessing some material.

Suggestion 1

Group Redux: If you liked the format of the group today, think of songs or scenes from movies or shows that make you feel a particular way.

1._____

2._____

3._____

Suggestion 2

Imaginal: You could spend time writing down a story of something that happened to you that made you feel a particularly strong emotion that you might try to avoid or escape. Your story could usefully be about food, eating, or body image, although it doesn't have to be, and it should be something that you can remember in good detail, particularly how you felt at that time. Try to remember a story that will make you feel a little uncomfortable so that you can become aware of these feelings and begin to tolerate them. You are going to use this piece of writing as your mood induction. Use Form 10.1: Mood Induction Recording to observe your emotions after you've written and read through your story.

Homework

Many of the forms and worksheets will need to be filled out more than once. We are including one blank copy of every worksheet and form for you. For those items that you will need more than once, your therapist will provide additional copies, or you can download blank copies yourself from the TreatmentsThatWork™ website at www.oxfordclinicalpsych.com/UTforEDs.

- Fill out Form 3.1: Eating, Depression, and Anxiety (EDA).
- Plot scores on Form 3.2: EDA Graph.

- Fill out Form 4.1: Regular Eating Food Log.
- Complete Form 8.1: The ARC of Emotional Experiences.
- Mood Induction Homework (suggestion 1 or 2).
- Fill out Form 10.1: Mood Induction Recording.
- Read Chapter 11 and preview the exercises.

Form 10.1
Mood Induction Recording

Use this form to record what you noticed. Rate the intensity of your emotion 0 to 8, with 0 = not at all, 4 = moderately, 8 = extremely.

Stimuli (Images, Video, Music)	Primary Emotional Response	Intensity (0–10)	Secondary Emotional Responses	Intensity (0–10)
	Emotion: Thoughts Physical Sensations Behaviors and Impulses		Emotions: Thoughts Physical Sensations Behaviors and Impulses	
	Emotion: Thoughts Physical Sensations Behaviors and Impulses		Emotions: Thoughts Physical Sensations Behaviors and Impulses	

Cognitive Flexibility

Automatic Thoughts and Thinking Traps

CHAPTER 11

GOALS

- Understand automatic thoughts, which are fast, subjective interpretations of the world.
  - Automatic thoughts influence and are influenced by emotion.
  - There can be more than one interpretation of a situation.
  - Cognitive flexibility means being able to consider various interpretations.
- Understand how thinking traps influence thoughts to produce negative emotion:
  - Jumping to conclusions, or probability overestimation
  - Thinking the worst, or catastrophizing

HOMEWORK REVIEW

- Fill out Form 3.1: Eating, Depression, and Anxiety (EDA).
- Plot scores on Form 3.2: EDA Graph.
- Fill out Form 4.1: Regular Eating Food Log.
- Complete Form 8.1: The ARC of Emotional Experiences.
- Mood Induction Homework (suggestion 1 or 2).
- Fill out Form 10.1: Mood Induction Recording.

There are two technical words to know for this session: cognitions and appraisals. *Cognition* is just a technical word for thinking and thoughts. *Appraisals* are the meanings that we make of things—how we interpret or understand the very complicated world around us.

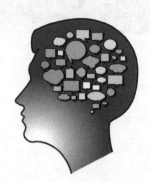

We have thousands of cognitions, or thoughts, every day. Some of them we really pay attention to, and some of them we allow to pass by. Think of watching clouds. Did you ever lie on the ground and look for cloud animals or shapes and figures in the clouds? When you stare up at the cloudy sky, you probably see that there are many clouds floating up there, but you will perhaps choose to focus on only a few.

If we decide that a particular cloud has the shape of an animal, that is an interpretation, also known as an appraisal. We cannot focus on every single thought, and we cannot take the time to make a new meaning or interpretation of every single piece of the world. So, we make automatic appraisals many times a day. We need this shortcut to efficiently operate in the world.

These automatic appraisals are typically happening outside of our awareness. However, as you can imagine, our emotions really have a powerful impact on how we interpret any given situation or what we think about that situation. If you're having a really good day, you will view the world through a cheery lens. Alternatively, if you're having a really bad day, you may interpret the things people say or do in a more negative way. Your mood affects your thoughts, and then your thoughts affect your mood in turn.

In therapy, you will hopefully gain a greater awareness of the ways that your personal appraisals affect your mood and behavior. You can develop flexibility in your appraisals by first identifying automatic appraisals that are unhelpful, and then learning to generate alternative appraisals or interpretations, a skill we call *cognitive reappraisal*.

Here are three important ideas when it comes to appraisals:

1. There is a reciprocal relationship between your thoughts and your emotions. How you interpret or appraise situations affects your emotions, and also your emotions influence your thoughts.

2. Your appraisal of a situation or experience can vary depending on which part of it you focus on. There are usually a number of different ways in which the situation as a whole can be interpreted or appraised.

3. Your appraisal of a situation or experience can vary depending on how much meaning you assign to a situation or experience. If a situation is important to you, and your emotional reaction is strong, your automatic appraisal may feel very believable, and you may be less flexible in considering another interpretation.

To put these three ideas into motion let's consider, for instance, that you just made a presentation in class or at work. If your teacher or boss pointed out something you could improve on:

- You might interpret this as indicating failure: "Because my teacher pointed out I could improve my eye contact, I must have blown that presentation."

- Or you might interpret the feedback as constructive criticism: "The presentation went OK. Next time I can make it even better by improving my eye contact."

- You might select the criticism to focus on instead of all the positive comments that were made. If the presentation was extremely important to you, you might take this perceived failure to mean something about you as a person: "I really blew that presentation. I am such a failure!"

- Or, alternatively, you could look at it as a single event: "This presentation didn't go so well, but I will do better next time."

This is the way that the human mind works—serving as a filter by focusing on certain aspects of a situation, assigning meaning to those aspects, and thus increasing the efficiency and speed with which we can respond to a given situation. This process can be helpful, and we will look at this idea in more detail in our closing discussion. We also tend to draw on our experiences from the past to 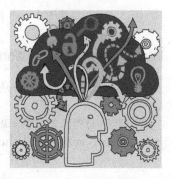 help us interpret or appraise current situations, and we often use these interpretations and appraisals to project what might happen in the future. As you can imagine, these different appraisals will have quite different consequences for our emotions, including what we do and how we feel.

In-Session Exercise 11.1
Flexibility with Appraisals

Here's an exercise to help illustrate the ideas that appraisals are subjective and that they are influenced by emotions, situations, and experience.

Take a moment to look at the picture on the next page. Think about what might be happening in the picture, and then fill out the Interpretations Activity Worksheet.

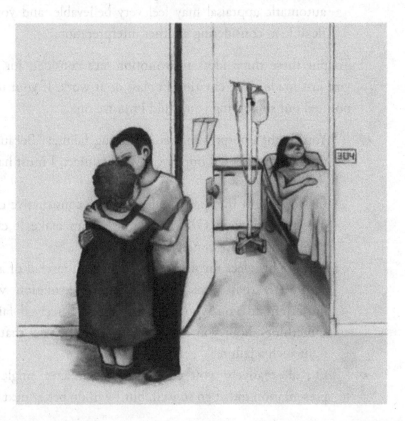

Used with permission from Oxford University Press

Interpretations Activity Worksheet

Remember, there are no "right answers," even if some of the appraisals might seem right.

What were your <u>automatic</u> interpretations about the picture? (These are the first things that jumped into your mind about what's happening in the picture.)

_____

_____

_____

_____

What factors contributed to your automatic interpretations (e.g., past experiences, memories, specific aspects you focused on in the picture, etc.)?

_____

_____

_____

_____

Generate some _alternative_ interpretations about what the picture might mean (come up with at least three alternatives). If your first, automatic interpretation was a negative one, see if you can come up with a positive interpretation. If your first, automatic interpretation was positive, see if you can come up with a negative interpretation. Practice being flexible with your interpretations.

_____

_____

_____

_____

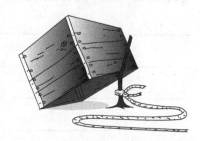

When we find ourselves stuck in patterns where our first impressions are usually negative, we may be falling into a thinking trap. To show what we mean, let's go back to the example of having given a presentation in class or at work. Imagine that after you received some criticism, you became very upset. Let's imagine that your thoughts about the presentation, yourself, and your job, were along the lines of "My boss/teacher thought that was terrible," "I'm going to get a bad job review/grade in the class," and "I might even lose my job/flunk out of school!" Those thoughts would probably make you feel terrible. Let's see how they might reflect common thinking traps.

Jumping to conclusions, or probability overestimation

This is when you overestimate the likelihood of negative events happening. With limited evidence except for your emotional   state, you assume there will be a bad outcome. Similarly, you may ignore evidence that would suggest another, perhaps equally likely, outcome. These traps make our appraisals more rigid and less flexible, which can keep us stuck in the cycle of strong emotions.

Can you see any ways that the thoughts about the presentation, discussed earlier, reflect jumping to conclusions?

Thinking the worst, or catastrophizing

This is when you automatically predict that the *worst possible* scenario is going to happen, without considering other possible outcomes. You also tend to underestimate your ability to cope with this outcome if it should occur. This thinking trap can keep us stuck on one particular interpretation, fueling the intensity of our emotional response and preventing us from adopting a more flexible, realistic perspective.

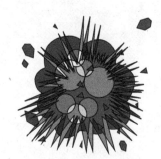

Can you see any ways that the thoughts about the presentation, discussed earlier, reflect catastrophizing?

Thinking traps usually make us feel bad in some way, and they usually occur in emotionally provocative situations. It can be *so* difficult, but before cannonballing into these situations and reacting with strong emotion, we are going to practice considering whether there are alternative possible interpretations of the situation. We call this *cognitive reappraisal*, and it's one way to get out of these thinking traps. When we re-evaluate or reappraise our initial interpretations (automatic appraisals) of a situation, we try to look at them not as "truths" but rather as one of many possible ways to interpret the situation.

Keep in mind that we want to practice identifying thinking traps and developing cognitive flexibility in a *nonjudgmental way*. The point is not to think, "I am so stupid for falling into this trap" or to punish yourself for having that thought. And we have all had people say to us, "Just don't look at it that way!" or "You are looking at it wrong!" These patterns have come about for a reason—it is not your "fault" you think this way, and you aren't doing anything wrong. These patterns are also pretty difficult to change. So try not to listen to judgmental voices—your own, or those of others. Rather, we want to practice becoming aware of the trap, knowing the way your mind works, and considering the possible trap within the context of the emotion you are experiencing, as *one way* of thinking about the situation. Remember that we don't make negative automatic appraisals all the time—just particularly in situations that are highly emotional, and/or ones that are very influenced by our prior experiences.

How do we become more flexible in our thinking?

Here are some questions that you can ask yourself to begin developing cognitive flexibility in situations that bring up strong emotions and strong automatic thoughts. These questions, which will also appear in Worksheet 11.1, will help you to re-evaluate jumping to conclusions and to "decatastrophize" catastrophic thoughts.

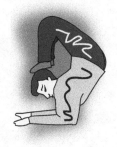

Questions for negative automatic thoughts

Use these questions when you notice yourself falling into a thinking trap:

- Do I know for certain that this thought will happen or is true?
- What evidence do I have for and against this thought or belief?
- Has this happened in the past every single time I've been in a similar situation?
- If it has happened in the past, could there be another explanation for that?
- How much does it feel like this is true? What is a more realistic chance that it is true?
- Could my thought be influenced by the intense emotions I'm experiencing now?
- If it were true, could I cope with it? How would I actually handle it?
- Even if it were true, could I live with it?

In-Session Exercise 11.2
Cognitive Flexibility Exercise

This part of the exercise will get you started. You will have to finish the rest of the activity for homework, and review it in the next session. For this part of the exercise you will need:

- Form 8.1: The ARC of Emotional Experiences
- A pen or pencil
- Worksheet 11.2: Re-evaluating Automatic Appraisals, found later in this chapter

First, fill out the ARC form for a recent intense emotional experience.

Next, using the two descriptions of common thinking traps, see if you can find a good example of probability overestimation and/or catastrophizing that fits into the ARC. Remember, it's not crucial that you identify the exact right type of thinking trap for the thought on your ARC; rather, the purpose is to begin to recognize when you are falling into these rigid ways of appraising situations, so that you take the next step in treatment: increasing flexibility in your thinking.

Next, put your ARC side by side with Worksheet 11.2: Re-evaluating Automatic Appraisals. Then take your example from your ARC and write it in the appraisals column, along with the antecedent (what happened before the emotion), the emotion(s), and the thinking trap. Then stop.

If there is time left in this current session, let's get started working together to reappraise these automatic appraisals using Worksheet 11.2.

Homework

Many of the forms and worksheets will need to be filled out more than once. We are including one blank copy of every worksheet and form for you. For those items that you will need more than once, your therapist will provide additional copies, or you can download blank copies yourself from the TreatmentsThatWork™ website at www.oxfordclinicalpsych.com/UTforEDs.

- Fill out Form 3.1: Eating, Depression, and Anxiety (EDA).
- Plot scores on Form 3.2: EDA Graph.
- Fill out Form 4.1: Regular Eating Food Log.
- Complete Form 8.1: The ARC of Emotional Experiences.
- Read and complete Worksheet 11.1: Cognitive Reappraisal Strategies.
- Finish filling out Worksheet 11.2: Re-evaluating Automatic Appraisals.
- Read and complete Worksheet 11.3: Obsessive Thoughts.
- Read Chapter 12 and preview the exercises.

Worksheet 11.1
Cognitive Reappraisal Strategies

Countering probability overestimation: learning to re-evaluate jumping to conclusions

The first cognitive reappraisal skill is *countering probability overestimation*, or learning how to re-evaluate jumping to conclusions. After identifying the automatic appraisal, the next step is to realistically examine the probability of that outcome actually happening. Essentially, you want to look for evidence from the past or present to test how likely it is that your belief/fear will actually come true. Use these questions when you notice yourself falling into a thinking trap:

1. Do I know for certain that _____ will happen?
2. Am I 100% sure these awful consequences will occur?
3. What evidence do I have for this fear or belief?
4. What happened in the past in this type of situation?
5. Do I have a crystal ball? How can I be sure that I know the answer?
6. Could there be any other explanations?
7. How much does it feel like _____ will happen?
8. What is the true likelihood that _____ will happen?
9. Is my negative prediction driven by the intense emotions I'm experiencing?
10. Is _____ really so important or consequential?

Decatastrophizing: learning to re-evaluate thinking the worst

The second cognitive reappraisal skill is *decatastrophizing*, or learning to re-evaluate thinking the worst. Once you have identified the core automatic appraisal, the next step is to realistically examine the evidence based on how you have coped in the past if something similar has occurred.

1. What is the worst that could happen? How bad is that?
2. Has _____ ever happened in the past?
   a. If yes, how did you cope with it? How did you handle it?
   b. If no, how do you think you'd cope with it or handle it now?
3. If it did happen—so what?
4. Even if _____ happens, can you live through it?
5. Is _____ really so terrible?

Worksheet 11.2

Re-evaluating Automatic Appraisals

SITUATION/TRIGGER	AUTOMATIC APPRAISAL(s)	EMOTION(s)	IDENTIFY THINKING TRAP	GENERATE ALTERNATIVE APPRAISALS

Worksheet 11.3
Obsessive Thoughts

Evaluating obsessive, intrusive, nonsensical thoughts

Sometimes people have thoughts that seem to just come into their mind and don't make sense. This is quite common and happens to most people. Whereas most people are able to let these sorts of "strange" thoughts go, maybe by telling themselves, "That was weird!" and then forgetting about them, others might get "stuck" in the thoughts. For some, the thoughts are intrusive and distressing, and they can't seem to block them out of their mind. For example, someone might be bothered by an intrusive thought that she will harm someone she loves or that she might do something terrible. These types of intrusive thoughts are also experienced as "automatic," but they are a little different from what we have been discussing so far. The types of thoughts we are discussing here do not make sense and can be very difficult to challenge.

The reality is that the obsessive, intrusive, nonsensical thought is not what needs to be reappraised. *Instead, what needs to be evaluated is our interpretation of what having this thought might mean.*

If you are having these types of thoughts, ask yourself, "How does having this thought make me feel? What do I think having this thought means?" The interpretation a person has about intrusive, nonsensical thoughts is what makes these thoughts distressing to one person and not to another. One person might have horrible intrusive thoughts and be able to "shake them off" as having no real meaning about who that person is or what that person might do. Others, however, can have the same thought and interpret the thought as meaning something terrible about themselves or as something they will inevitably act on. Some common interpretations that can be very distressing—but can be shown not to be true—are "These thoughts mean I am crazy," "These thoughts mean I am evil," or "These thoughts mean I will do something destructive to myself or someone I love."

It is the interpretation of what these thoughts mean that is the source of distress, and it is here that the strategies discussed in this chapter should be used. If you are having these types of intrusive thoughts, see if you can identify your automatic appraisals about these intrusive thoughts, and see if you can generate some alternative appraisals using the skills discussed earlier.

If you have obsessional thoughts, make a note of them, take it to your therapist, and try to identify what the meaning is that you make of the fact that you have these thoughts.

_____

_____

_____

_____

_____

- Understand what core beliefs are and where they come from.
- See the relationship between negative core beliefs and negative automatic thoughts.
- Learn the downward arrow technique to identify negative core beliefs.

- Fill out Form 3.1: Eating, Depression, and Anxiety (EDA).
- Plot scores on Form 3.2: EDA Graph.
- Fill out Form 4.1: Regular Eating Food Log.
- Complete Form 8.1: The ARC of Emotional Experiences.
- Read and complete Worksheet 11.1: Cognitive Reappraisal Strategies.
- Finish filling out Worksheet 11.2: Re-evaluating Automatic Appraisals.
- Read and complete Worksheet 11.3: Obsessive Thoughts.
- Read Chapter 12 and preview the exercises.

Core beliefs

Core beliefs are powerful. They exist deep within our brains, and they influence how we think. They are at the root, or the core, of your automatic thoughts about yourself. As we mentioned, they can be positive or negative. The thoughts component of our emotions may often contain an automatic thought, and underlying this thought is the core belief. Figure 12.1 illustrates two main ways that core beliefs form.

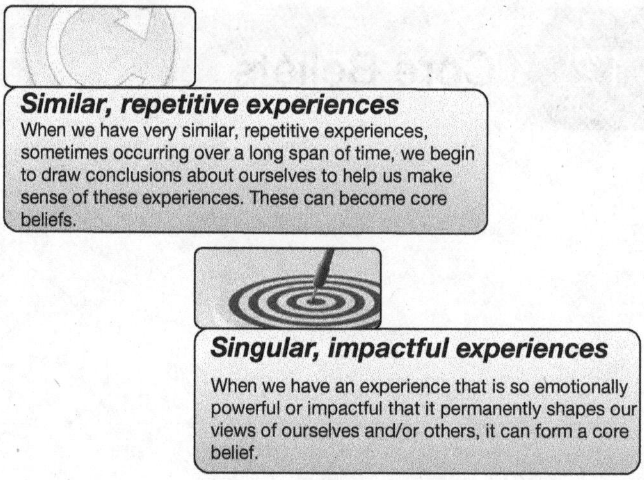

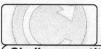

Similar, repetitive experiences

When we have very similar, repetitive experiences, sometimes occurring over a long span of time, we begin to draw conclusions about ourselves to help us make sense of these experiences. These can become core beliefs.

Singular, impactful experiences

When we have an experience that is so emotionally powerful or impactful that it permanently shapes our views of ourselves and/or others, it can form a core belief.

Figure 12.1:

How Core Beliefs Form

Similar, repetitive experiences

When we have multiple similar, repetitive experiences, we come up with a general appraisal (core belief) about ourselves and/or the world that "fits" with these experiences.

Let's imagine that during high school there was a particular subject that you consistently failed on your tests, no matter how hard you tried. This difficult and defeating experience may form the core belief "I am a failure" or "I'm a disappointment to my parents." Although this is a sad thought, it helped you make sense of what was happening. Unfortunately, because it was a core belief, it also helped explain away or even predict future disappointments. Let's say that you sat for an exam with the understanding "I am a failure" and "I am a disappointment to my parents." What would the outcomes be?

- Do you think you would be surprised and disappointed if you received a low grade?
- What else would you think?
- What would this repetitive experience help you to conclude?
- How would this influence your immediate *and* future behavior?

Someone with childhood diabetes, which requires careful medical monitoring and treatment, may have the core belief "I am defective" or "I could die easily." A survivor of chronic child abuse may carry the core belief "I deserve to be punished" or "I am in danger."

Singular, impactful experiences

Even a short-lived experience or an isolated occurrence can leave its mark on your deepest beliefs about yourself. For example, a wife who learns, after 15 years of marriage, that her husband is having an affair may conclude, "I am not good enough." Or perhaps in middle school, when you were forming ideas about your social identity, one cruel thing that was said to you could lead you to conclude that "other people don't like me."

- What could some of the outcomes here be?
- How would this influence your immediate *and* future behavior?
- Do you think negative core beliefs occurring in a specific event can generalize to other events in life?

Core beliefs: the root of the issue

Imagine that an automatic thought is a plant; then the roots of the plant are the core belief from which it sprouted. The core belief influences how we see things and interpret things. As humans, we pay attention to things in our world that are congruent with (that agree with) our inner world. What that means is that you are more likely to pay attention to and remember things that confirm your core beliefs. It's as if you are viewing the world through a pair of tinted lenses that make certain things stand out for you and others harder to see.

Now let's imagine you are the high school student who consistently failed tests, and your therapist or dietitian suggests that you have to add more foods to your diet. Your automatic thoughts might be, "I have been eating wrong; my therapist is

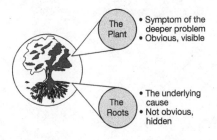

disappointed in me" or "There is no way I am going to be able to do this task—it's impossible." In the context of what you've been through, your appraisal about not being able to change your diet makes sense, given how you view yourself and your ability to do hard things.

Here are a few other examples:

- If you begin to feel short of breath, you may think, "I'm going to have a panic attack."
- If you see a peer in the hallway who looks at you without smiling, your immediate thought may be "She's mad at me" or even "She doesn't like me."

The core beliefs that underlie these automatic thoughts or immediate thoughts are deeply rooted through our experiences over time. In these examples, the core beliefs could be "The world isn't safe," or "I'll always be alone," or "I'm not a likeable person."

In-Session Exercise 12.1
The Downward Arrow

We're going to spend the remaining time today doing the downward arrow. The downward arrow technique is both an emotional exposure and an awareness tool. The function of this tool is to bring about insight and facilitate new learning, which may not be a feel-good experience at first. In fact, if it brings up strong emotion, you are probably identifying important core beliefs.

Turn to Form 12.1: Downward Arrow at the end of this chapter. We take a surface-level thought, or appraisal, and ask ourselves a question: "And *so what* if this were true?" This helps us understand why the thought is important and meaningful to us, and it provides us with a new thought to explore, to which we can ask: "What would happen next?" or "If this were true, what would it mean about me?" In so doing, we get to an underlying thought or belief, and we explore this thought the same way. As we repeat this process, we "follow the arrow down" and deepen the intensity of the emotional experience with every layer. We eventually arrive at a core belief.

Rolling with the content

As you can see, there are several questions from which we can choose to pull in the service of exploring the thought. Remember, the goal is to uncover a more personally relevant and emotionally evocative thought. The follow-up question that is used each time may be different, based on what the content of the thought is and what makes the most sense. For example:

- If this were true, what would it mean about me?
- Why does this matter to me?
- What would happen if this were true?
- What would happen next?
- What does this mean about how people would perceive me?

There are common automatic thoughts that reflect different core beliefs. You can choose one listed here to work on with the downward arrow, or come up with your own automatic (negative or anxious) thoughts from the past week. Use the questions above to get to your core beliefs using Form 12.1: Downward Arrow.

Common automatic thoughts (create your own variation!) are as follows:

- If I eat _____, I am going to _____ (get fat, binge eat, etc.).
- If I _____, I am going to be uncomfortable and embarrass myself.
- If I _____, then _____ is going to judge me.

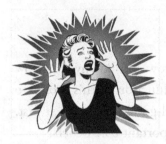

You may be wondering, "What now?!" when you get to the core belief. Perhaps you even thought, "Well, that made me feel worse!" If you thought similar thoughts, then you're on the right track—we can't work through these feelings until we get to them!

First, just sit with it for a minute. Let yourself identify what feelings it brings up. Think a little about where you think that core belief might have come from. To start exercising flexible thinking, see if any of these approaches might help when you run up against a core belief:

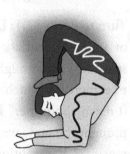

- "I'm doing it again! This is an automatic thought based on past things in my life."
- "Yes, it might feel that way, that's how it has been for me in my life, but that doesn't mean I'm *certain* to fail."
- "This is my core belief I carry with me that's based on my past, not this current experience/challenge."
- "This is a thinking trap! I am underestimating my ability to cope with the situation. Let me see if I can find a reappraisal in this moment."

Many of the forms and worksheets will need to be filled out more than once. We are including one blank copy of every worksheet and form for you. For those items that you will need more than once, your therapist will provide additional copies, or you can download blank copies yourself from the TreatmentsThatWork™ website at www.oxfordclinicalpsych.com/UTforEDs.

- Fill out Form 3.1: Eating, Depression, and Anxiety (EDA).
- Plot scores on Form 3.2: EDA Graph.
- Fill out Form 4.1: Regular Eating Food Log.
- Complete Form 8.1: The ARC of Emotional Experiences.
- Before the next session, try to complete one Form 12.1: Downward Arrow *each day* for different emotions and automatic thoughts that come up.
- Read Chapter 13 and preview the exercises.

FORM 12.1
Downward Arrow

Automatic Appraisal: _____

If this were true, what would it mean about me? Why does this matter to me?
What would happen if this were true? What would happen next?

Underlying Appraisal: _____

If this were true, what would it mean about me? Why does this matter to me?
What would happen if this were true? What would happen next?

Underlying Appraisal: _____

If this were true, what would it mean about me? Why does this matter to me?
What would happen if this were true? What would happen next?

Underlying Appraisal: _____

If this were true, what would it mean about me? Why does this matter to me?
What would happen if this were true? What would happen next?

Underlying Appraisal: _____

Behavioral Flexibility

GOALS

- Understand how suppression of thoughts and emotions can be counterproductive.
  - Try thought suppression exercise to demonstrate this idea.
- Identify three types of avoidance:
  - Behavioral avoidance (obvious and subtle)
  - Cognitive avoidance
  - Safety signals

HOMEWORK REVIEW

- Fill out Form 3.1: Eating, Depression, and Anxiety (EDA).
- Plot scores on Form 3.2: EDA Graph.
- Fill out Form 4.1: Regular Eating Food Log.
- Complete Form 8.1: The ARC of Emotional Experiences.
- Before the next session, try to complete one Form 12.1: Downward Arrow each day for different emotions and automatic thoughts that come up.
- Read Chapter 13 and preview the exercises.

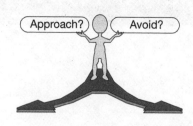

The key concept for this session is emotion avoidance. *Emotion avoidance* means any strategies we use to avoid feeling strong emotions or to prevent our emotions from becoming more intense. Although these responses may be useful in some situations, they rarely work well in the long term and they can even increase the intensity of our emotions when we encounter a similar situation in the future. In this session you will develop greater awareness of your own patterns of emotion avoidance and prepare to challenge these responses through emotion exposures.

Emotion-driven behaviors (EDBs) are a strategy of emotion escape. Strong emotions can drive us to engage in specific behaviors sometimes before we even have a chance to think about it. This can be helpful and adaptive, for instance when we are in immediate danger (e.g., seeing a bear in the woods). However, sometimes EDBs are not consistent with the situation at hand (e.g., having the same response when we see a plate of spaghetti, or when we are asked a question by our boss, as we would when seeing a bear in the woods). These same avoidant behaviors, while relieving us from the experience of intense or uncomfortable emotions in the short term, can actually limit our lives in important ways, or even be harmful.

Today we will be talking mostly about avoidance as a general concept, why it doesn't work, and the different kinds of avoidance that we might engage in. In this session, we are going to focus on the *avoidance*, which is what happens when we *anticipate* emotion coming and try to avoid feeling it. In the next session, we will be talking about emotion-driven behaviors, meaning the *behaviors*, like binge eating, purging, or physically escaping, that we engage in *after* we are feeling an emotion, in order to get away from that emotion. The same behavior can be avoidance in one situation and an emotion-driven behavior in another, just depending on *when* it occurs in the process of having an emotional experience. A simple way to remember the difference is that emotion avoidance comes before the emotion and emotion-driven behaviors come after. Some behaviors belong in both categories, so don't worry about the distinction too much.

One way that people attempt to control their emotional experiences is through emotion avoidance. Emotion avoidance is when we engage in behaviors (do things) designed to *prevent ourselves* from experiencing strong or unwanted emotions. For example, someone who has found elevators frightening might decide to take the stairs from now on. Some people with body image problems might avoid going to the beach, because they are afraid how they would feel if people saw their body. Some people with social anxiety will avoid social gatherings or public places. Emotion avoidance most often occurs with regard to negative emotions, but it can occur for positive emotions as well. For instance, some people suffering from depression report difficulty in allowing themselves to feel positive emotions—maybe due to fear of disappointment, or because happiness feels unfamiliar and strange. In order to have an example to work with, think of and share a situation or thing that you avoid because it causes emotions that you don't want to have.

What is the problem with avoidance?

If avoidance worked really well to manage our emotions, then there wouldn't be a problem. Actually it does serve a purpose in the short term—if we are able to avoid the emotion that we find distressing, then why not? The problem is that over the long term, chronic avoidance causes problems in a number of ways:

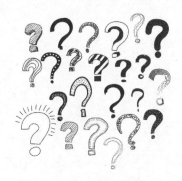

- **Avoidance often doesn't really work.**
  It temporarily decreases an emotion, but it can't make it go away.
- When we habitually avoid an emotion, **we never learn** that the emotion could be tolerable or that it would pass on its own without our efforts to avoid or escape.
- When we habitually avoid an emotion or the situation that provokes the emotion, **we give ourselves negative messages**—like "I can't handle that emotion" or "That situation is dangerous to me"—and this backfires to cause more fear or distress the next time we face a similar situation.
- This process can become **progressive over time**, so we have to avoid more and more situations and find the emotion more and more difficult to deal with. For example, someone with a fear of driving a

car might start with not driving on the highway, but then he finds the city starts to make him nervous, and finally he decides it is too scary to drive at all.

■ Some of the things we do to avoid emotions **really hurt us**, like eating symptoms, substance abuse, cutting, or suicidal gestures on the extreme side, and not being able to meet the demands of life or missing out on certain opportunities more subtly.

In-Session Exercise 13.1
Demonstration of Emotion Avoidance

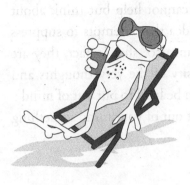

We're going to do a quick experiment that will help you understand the concept of emotion avoidance, and to see how emotion avoidance strategies work (and don't work!). Focus on the picture of the frog, and really take in the details of this picture for a few moments. Now close your eyes and follow these instructions, which your therapist will read aloud:

For about 1 minute, try to think about the frog. Don't think about anything else except the frog. [A minute passes.] Open your eyes. How successful were you in thinking about this creature?

*OK, now close your eyes again for another minute and think about anything you want to, but absolutely **do not** think about the frog. [A minute passes.] Open your eyes. What did you notice?*

The paradoxical effect of suppression

Essentially, when people are asked to *not* think about something, they actually become overly focused on it and cannot help but think about it. In-Session Exercise 13.1 illustrates the idea that attempts to suppress negative thoughts and emotions are often unsuccessful. In fact, they are likely to increase the frequency and intensity of the very thoughts and emotions you are trying to suppress. If it can be hard to put out of mind a sunbathing frog, think how hard it is to put out of your mind something that is actually really bothering you!

Three different types of avoidance

Some types of emotion avoidance are more obvious, such as when someone refuses to enter a situation that is likely to produce emotional distress. *Overt behavioral avoidance* is when you strongly believe that a situation will bring up a strong emotion that you do not wish to experience, and you consciously choose to avoid that situation. Examples include not going to restaurants that serve your feared foods, not eating in public, walking instead of using public transportation, not attending a party that would make you nervous, avoiding crowded areas, avoiding driving on the highway, and staying in bed.

There are other, less obvious things that people do to avoid their emotions. These subtle emotion avoidance strategies can be broken down into three types: subtle behavioral avoidance, cognitive avoidance, and the use of safety signals.

Subtle behavior avoidance

Subtle behavioral avoidance typically happens when a person enters a situation that they associate with intense emotions, and full escape from the situation is not an option. As a result, the person may engage in a variety of subtle behaviors of which they may not even be 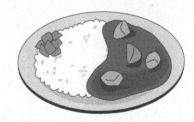 fully aware to prevent the feared emotion from getting stronger. For example, if you are anxious about certain foods that you have to eat, you might keep them further away on the plate or try to avoid fully tasting them. If you are afraid of feelings associated with your body appearance, then you might keep your eyes averted from mirrors or angle yourself a certain way when you take pictures. People who are nervous about social interaction often don't make eye contact and they talk softly, fold their arms, put their hands in their pockets, or avoid disagreeing with other people.

Cognitive avoidance strategies

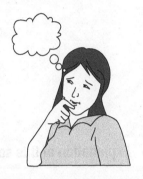

Cognitive avoidance strategies are often difficult to identify, and you may not even be aware that you are using them. The word "cognitive" here refers to anything you do to avoid having to think about, remember, or pay attention to something that is distressing. Some common examples of cognitive avoidance strategies are *distraction* (e.g., reading a book, listening to music, watching television) and *tuning out* (e.g., pretending you are not in the situation or not fully engaging in the experience of being in the situation). Distraction might seem useful because it keeps our minds from running away, but this can also be a form of emotion avoidance. People with eating disorders often do this when they are trying to eat—they try to think about anything except the food going into their bodies. As another example, someone who worries about the safety of loved ones may watch television or keep busy when their loved ones go out at night. The person is fearful that if they don't distract themself and prevent negative thoughts and feelings, they'll become overwhelmed by their anxiety and worry. Even reassuring yourself too much can be an avoidance strategy—just insisting that "it's going to be fine" can be a way to pretend or to avoid being worried or sad.

Safety signals

When someone is unable to directly avoid an emotionally provoking situation and they are afraid that cognitive avoidance strategies will not be sufficient, they may come to rely on safety signals. *Safety signals* are any items that people carry with them that they think will make them feel comfortable or calm them in times of extreme

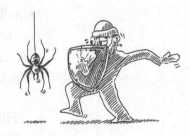

distress, despite the fact that these items may lack any real usefulness in dealing with a potentially threatening experience. Thus, safety signals can have almost a magical or superstitious quality to them and can function sort of like a talisman. Some common examples of safety signals are water bottles, medication (or even empty medication bottles), cellphones, certain pieces of clothing, or dolls or stuffed animals. Sometimes the safety signal can be another person. The presence of the object may feel calming in the short term, but it can also reinforce the idea that uncomfortable, unexpected emotional experiences are unmanageable and overwhelming by sending the message that the only way you can cope with these experiences is by having your safety signal with you. It may be time to ditch your lucky socks, clean out your pocketbook, and work toward facing situations, and accompanying emotions, head on.

Explanation of this session's homework

The homework is to identify some avoidance strategies that you engage in and choose some that you are going to try to stop doing. It is even more helpful and informative to try to do the opposite of avoidance. In each case, the "opposite action" is going to depend on what the avoidance behavior is. We should take a look at Worksheet 13.2: Reducing Avoidance and Form 13.1: Reducing Avoidance Practice Chart in the session to make sure it makes sense to you. You have to remember that when you first stop doing them you may feel an upsurge in anxiety because you have come to depend on these things. But as you persist, you will find that the anxiety associated with the issue overall will start to come down.

Homework

Many of the forms and worksheets will need to be filled out more than once. We are including one blank copy of every worksheet and form for you. For those items that you will need more than once, your therapist will provide additional copies, or you can download blank copies yourself from the TreatmentsThatWork™ website at www.oxfordclinicalpsych.com/UTforEDs.

- Fill out Form 3.1: Eating, Depression, and Anxiety (EDA).
- Plot scores on Form 3.2: EDA Graph.
- Fill out Form 4.1: Regular Eating Food Log.

- Complete Form 8.1: The ARC of Emotional Experiences.
- Review Table 13.1: Example of a List of Emotion Avoidance Strategies, and then fill out Worksheet 13.1: List of Emotion Avoidance Strategies.
- Complete Worksheet 13.2: Reducing Avoidance.
- Complete Form 13.1: Reducing Avoidance Practice Chart.
- Read Chapter 14 and preview the exercises.

Table 13.1 Example of a List of Emotion Avoidance Strategies

Subtle Behavioral Avoidance	Cognitive Avoidance Strategies	Safety Signals
BODY IMAGE Not look in reflective surfaces (windows, mirrors, etc.) Wear baggy and/or black clothing Keep my gaze away from my legs when I'm sitting down Never look at myself when I'm naked Don't go to swimming pools or public changing rooms FOOD AND EATING Not eating certain foods Not allowing myself to get full Chew for a long time Eat small bites Postpone eating as long as possible Look away from the plate GENERAL Procrastination Avoiding anything that can remind me of the past Keeping my phone on silent so I am not stressed out	Think about something else when I am being weighed, chat with the nurse Pretend I just don't have a body at all—that I don't exist from the neck down Imagine in really great detail how I will exercise when I get out of here Be a robot and eat without thinking Talk a lot with the people at the table Try not to think about the calories Singing that song over and over in my head Worry, obsessively plan for disaster Force myself to "think positive"	That one pair of yoga pants and the college sweatshirt Carrying Gas-X pills The picture of my sister Calling my mom every morning Having a water bottle with me Wearing earplugs when I go to sleep All my colored pencils, eraser, and sharpener for homework Carrying my phone and two chargers Having reading materials or self-help materials always on hand Spanx

Worksheet 13.1
List of Emotion Avoidance Strategies

The purpose of this list is to begin to identify some of the subtle ways that you may attempt to avoid uncomfortable emotions. We often use subtle avoidance strategies when we have to go into situations that we would rather completely avoid. Examples include when people are eating, interacting with other people, and talking about things that upset them. In the Subtle Behavioral Avoidance column, list subtle avoidance behaviors that you do. In the Cognitive Avoidance Strategies column, list mental techniques of avoidance, such as distracting yourself or tuning out. Finally, in the Safety Signals column, list anything that you carry with you or on you to ward off bad feelings.

Subtle Behavioral Avoidance	Cognitive Avoidance Strategies	Safety Signals

Worksheet 13.2
Reducing Avoidance

One of the most important things you can do to advance your treatment is to choose to reduce avoidance. Most people can identify some avoidance that is habitual but that they could try to change if they think about it, mentally prepare themselves, and try hard to address when the situation comes along.

Choose a few of the avoidance strategies you identified in Worksheet 13.1, and identify how you could do the *opposite*. The most benefit comes from deliberately trying to do the *opposite* of avoiding, which is leaning into emotion, or approaching it, rather than avoiding it or trying to dampen it down. For example, if you often speak quietly, you might decide that when you are feeling nervous in sessions you are going to talk in a particularly loud and clear voice. Or if you notice that you often chat a lot through a meal to distract yourself, you can decide that you are going to be very quiet and focus on the experience of the food. Other examples:

Avoidance strategy: Being really agreeable with people when you're nervous
Opposite action: Disagreeing with one thing somebody says in a conversation
Avoidance strategy: Not looking at yourself when you're naked
Opposite action: Make sure to look at every part of yourself in the shower, for a while
Avoidance strategy: Taking small bites and chewing a long time
Opposite action: Taking large bites and chewing only until it's possible to swallow

On this page, identify three avoidance strategies you can try to reduce, and the opposite action to try instead.

(1) First avoidance strategy you are going to try to reduce:

_____

Opposite action to this avoidance strategy:

_____

(2) Second avoidance strategy you are going to try to reduce:

_____

Opposite action to this avoidance strategy:

_____

(3) Third avoidance strategy you are going to try to reduce:

_____

Opposite action to this avoidance strategy:

_____

Form 13.1
Reducing Avoidance Practice Chart

Record the times that you tried to do the opposite of your avoidance and how it went. (The first row is filled out as an example.)

Avoidance Strategy	Opposite Action	Reaction and Experience
Being quiet in class or hardly ever speaking up	Making a comment as soon as possible after class started in a louder voice. Making several comments over group.	The first time I talked in a particular class I felt my heart pounding and I sounded really loud. But by the end I felt actually much more comfortable and plugged in than ever before.

CHAPTER 14 — Countering Emotion-Driven Behaviors

GOALS

- Understand and identify emotion-driven behaviors (EDBs) intended to escape from emotion.
- Identify when and how these EDBs can become problematic.
- Prepare for homework to substitute opposite actions in place of problematic EDBs.

HOMEWORK REVIEW

- Fill out Form 3.1: Eating, Depression, and Anxiety (EDA).
- Plot scores on Form 3.2: EDA Graph.
- Fill out Form 4.1: Regular Eating Food Log.
- Complete Form 8.1: The ARC of Emotional Experiences.
- Review Table 13.1: Example of a List of Emotion Avoidance Strategies, and then fill out Worksheet 13.1: List of Emotion Avoidance Strategies.
- Complete Worksheet 13.2: Reducing Avoidance.
- Complete Form 13.1: Reducing Avoidance Practice Chart.
- Read Chapter 14 and preview the exercises.

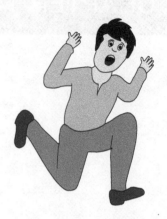

One very important aspect of emotions is that they tell us to act in a certain way or drive certain behaviors. For example, when we feel afraid, our tendency is to try to run away and escape—it's a natural response that protects us. As we discussed earlier, we refer to these responses as emotion-driven behaviors, or EDBs. EDBs are different from emotion avoidance in that EDBs happen in response to an emotion that has been triggered. Avoidance strategies, on the other hand, tend to happen *before* an emotion has had a chance to occur. Just like emotion avoidance, EDBs can become powerful habits in maintaining the cycle of emotions when the goal is to get away from the emotion.

For instance, the act of running away when we become really scared is an EDB meant to protect us from whatever is scaring us (flight, fight, or freeze response). **It is a behavior driven by the emotion itself.** Similarly, if something makes us very angry, the tendency will be to lash out, perhaps shout (or at the very least think about shouting) at whoever or whatever caused the offense, or, at the extreme, possibly physically attack the person in self-defense.

Our ability to respond quickly to our emotions to avoid threatening situations is necessary and adaptive (helpful). But in some situations, EDBs may not be entirely consistent with the current threat or may be less adaptive or even harmful to us in managing a particular situation. For instance, if you have a big presentation coming up at school or work that you need to prepare for, you might experience some anxiety that prompts you to prepare for the presentation. In this case, most people would agree that the behavior of preparing for the presentation is helpful in managing this situation. However, if you were to do a similar level of preparation for a social interaction with friends, we can see how this (overpreparation, in this case) might be a problem.

Another important aspect of human emotions is that they are often rooted in what has happened in the past, or what we think might happen in the future. Because we have the ability to think about the future or the past, our thoughts alone can often make us feel emotions without actually being triggered by anything happening in the present. Therefore, if we are responding to the emotions brought on by thoughts about a future or past event, this too can be considered an EDB.

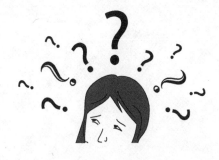

Try to identify if there are particular EDBs that you typically engage in or that are particularly problematic for you. Examples of EDBs are shown in Figure 14.1 and include:

- **Anxiety:** Someone becomes very worried about the safety of her family and frantically calls family members to see if they are all right.
- **Sadness:** Someone feels down and depressed and stays home for several days in a row to sleep instead of going to work, even though he knows there are supportive friends at work.
- **Fear:** Someone excessively washes her hands in response to feeling dirty or contaminated.
- **Anger:** Someone feels frustrated and angry over receiving a parking ticket. In response, he tears up the ticket and yells at the parking enforcement officer.

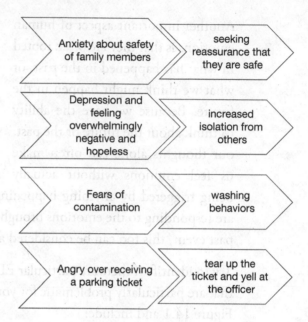

Anxiety about safety of family members	seeking reassurance that they are safe
Depression and feeling overwhelmingly negative and hopeless	increased isolation from others
Fears of contamination	washing behaviors
Angry over receiving a parking ticket	tear up the ticket and yell at the officer

Figure 14.1:

Examples of EDBs

How EDBs maintain the emotional response

Although EDBs are adaptive in certain situations, and they may reduce distressing emotions in the short term, they don't usually work in the long term. For example, Jordan begins writing a term paper but repeatedly stops (escape—an EDB) because writing the paper elicits strong depressive thoughts and emotions that drain her energy and motivation. Though this escape provides some relief in the short term, Jordan will probably feel even worse later because now she still has the same concerns about the paper with the additional pressure to write it in a short amount of time, and she may feel bad about herself for putting it off. Similarly, trying to make something perfect (which is one way of trying to establish control over a seemingly uncontrollable threatening situation) usually leads to higher and higher standards for work and more anxiety about additional tasks. In both cases, engaging in EDBs strengthens the connection between these situations and emotional experiences.

All behaviors are emotion-driven to some extent—we have different emotions, and our mind weighs our emotions in order to make decisions. We must figure out whether those decisions that we make are adaptive or not adaptive. Sometimes making a lot of improvements and focusing on perfection can seem to have some good outcomes and other times bad outcomes. In this treatment, we are more focused on EDBs that lead to the development of emotional disorders. As you are identifying which EDBs are problems for you, it is useful to think about all the different positive and negative outcomes.

Many people who feel negatively about their bodies decide to exercise more and eat healthy food because they think it will help to reduce those negative emotions. It is possible for those decisions to have good outcomes for some people at some times, but Figure 14.2 shows how these strategies can become problematic for people with an eating disorder (ED).

You can start to use these strategies to manage all your emotions. ED behaviors actually don't do a very good job of managing emotions that are about other situations.	If you only use those strategies—emotion-driven behaviors—they can become a self-perpetuating cycle.	You never learn other healthy ways of dealing with your emotions.
It is really difficult to feel that you have a "perfect" body or to keep up the effort that it takes.	When taken to an extreme, these behaviors have other negative consequences—your health, your concentration, your relationships, your mood—and these things make you feel more negative emotions, and so on. . .	Lots of new negative emotions come to be associated with not-dieting. New foods are scary. Failure is scary.

Figure 14.2:

Problems with Eating and Dieting Strategies to Manage Emotions

Identifying EDBs and developing opposite action tendencies

One way to begin changing current emotional responses with regard to intense emotions is to **adopt behaviors that promote a pattern of approach, as opposed to avoidance.** In other words, it is important to begin engaging in activities and

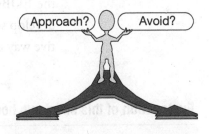

situations that are likely to evoke the emotions you are currently avoiding. In this way, you are able to gather more information about your ability to cope in any given situation. While you'll learn more about this in the next session, what are some situations that you are avoiding now that you want to work on approaching? Think about issues pertaining to food, to body image, or to anxiety or depression.

Research has found that one of the most effective ways to break the cycle of emotions and actually change the way you experience emotions is to do something that is completely different than what you would normally do in response to your

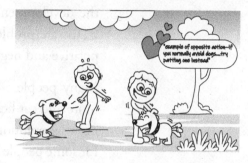

emotion. We refer to this as choosing an "opposite action," an **action that is opposite or counter to what you've done in the past in response to your emotions**. An opposite action doesn't always mean that you have to do something big—for example, it can be something like smiling instead of frowning when you're feeling down. Changing how you behave and respond can also change how you feel over time.

One point that is important to bring up here is that engaging in opposite *actions* (for example, smiling instead of frowning) is quite different from engaging in opposite *thoughts*. Trying to convince yourself that you are happy when you are down does not work. Trying to talk yourself into an emotion you don't have is an example of a cognitive avoidance strategy. What we are discussing here is doing different behaviors than those initially driven by the emotion (EDBs).

It may be helpful at this point to identify some of your typical EDBs and work on developing alternative behaviors. It's OK if you have trouble identifying some of the key ones at this point. You'll get a chance to work on identifying EDBs for homework. In session, start discussing some of the EDBs you would like to change as part of your treatment, and then develop some clear opposite actions that you believe will be a more adaptive way of responding to your emotions in the long term.

Explanation of this session's homework

Today for homework you have an EDB writing exercise, as well as two EDB forms to fill out, in addition to your usual EDAs. The instructions are clearly written on each homework assignment; however, we are going to go through the instructions before we leave today, so that you have an opportunity to clear up any questions that you may have. Take some time to add ideas about key EDBs and useful opposite actions in Worksheets 14.1: Identifying Your EDBs Writing Exercise and 14.2: Identifying Your

EDBs and Opposite Actions. You can write about them at more length for homework, but take some time in session to discuss whether you are on the right track. You will also be completing Form 14.1: Changing Your EDBs and Worksheet 14.3: EDB Reading and Reflection.

Homework

Many of the forms and worksheets will need to be filled out more than once. We are including one blank copy of every worksheet and form for you. For those items that you will need more than once, your therapist will provide additional copies, or you can download blank copies yourself from the TreatmentsThatWork™ website at www.oxfordclinicalpsych.com/UTforEDs.

- Fill out Form 3.1: Eating, Depression, and Anxiety (EDA).
- Plot scores on Form 3.2: EDA Graph.
- Fill out Form 4.1: Regular Eating Food Log.
- Complete Form 8.1: The ARC of Emotional Experiences.
- Complete Worksheet 14.1: Identifying Your EDBs Writing Exercise.
- Complete Worksheet 14.2: Identifying Your EDBs and Opposite Actions.
- Complete Form 14.1: Changing Your EDBs.
- Complete Worksheet 14.3: EDB Reading and Reflection.
- Read Chapter 15 and preview the exercises.

Instructions

To some extent, all of our behaviors are emotion-driven. When we think about what we should do next, our emotions help tell us whether our behavior will likely have a good or bad overall outcome. However, we aren't interested in examining all of our behaviors. We specifically want to take a look at EDBs that are problems for us—that are a part of our main emotional problems—and that seem to be a way of escaping an emotion we don't want to have. To help identify these EDBs, you might think about the following questions:

- What are your main emotional problems in life?
- What do you do as a part of these emotional problems that could be considered an EDB?
- Are there particular things that you do that are unhealthy?
- How could these unhealthy behaviors be driven by the desire to escape from or reduce particular emotions?

You are going to write about your own EDBs on the next page. You can read through this example to help you craft your own narrative:

Example

My main emotional problems are my eating disorder and my panic disorder. I also have a lot of pain associated with my divorce. As a part of my eating disorder, I exercise and restrict food because I am afraid of becoming fat. When I am feeling fat, or feeling threatened, I restrict food. I know when I am feeling stressed, I also eat less. I don't like feeling out of control, and I don't like feeling insecure, and I don't like feeling sad. Exercising and dieting helped me feel more in control, confident, and optimistic at one time.

As part of my panic disorder, I get really afraid of having panic attacks. When I start to feel panicky, I try to escape from any enclosed spaces or crowds. Running away is a big part of that. Sometimes I notice that I ask people for different kinds of help or reassurance because I'm afraid I'm going to have a panic attack, or I am sick, or that people can tell I am panicky and are judging me. So I might ask people if it is OK if I leave, or if it feels like my heart is beating really hard, if they think that could be a heart attack, or if they can see my hand shaking, and do they think that is crazy.

I think that EDBs contributed to my divorce in a lot of ways. I really didn't want to give up my eating disorder because that seemed overwhelming, so I pushed my husband away and got angry when he noticed what was going on. When I started to feel guilty about what I was doing with my husband, somehow that drove me to do it even more. It is really complicated. The divorce itself made me feel sad, guilty, angry, worthless—so many different bad things. I have been using my eating disorder to try make these emotions go away. I also avoid thinking about or talking about the divorce itself, or how it really makes me feel.

_____

_____

_____

_____

_____

_____

_____

_____

_____

_____

_____

_____

_____

_____

_____

_____

_____

_____

_____

_____

_____

_____

_____

_____

_____

_____

_____

Worksheet 14.2
Identifying Your EDBs and Opposite Actions

Recent, frequent, and problematic EDBs and possible opposite actions

The next part of the homework is to make a list of key EDBs that are parts of your emotional problems, and list some ideas for how you can do alternative opposite actions. Remember, there can be a lot of problems with EDBs—they can become automatic, they don't usually work, they teach you that you can't deal with your emotions, they teach you that emotions are dangerous, they tend to make the emotions stronger over time, and so on. Even if it isn't clear what the direct positive result would be of turning them around, if you know that they are a part of your emotional issues, then it is probably a good idea to try to reverse them. The first row is filled out as an example.

EDBs What is the action? What is the emotional situation?	Opposite Action
Dieting or exercising after I have talked to my ex-husband. Raging at him. Ignoring how sad I really feel.	Talking to a friend or writing in my journal about how I feel when I talk to him. Trying not to focus too much on my anger (which may be a secondary reaction) but really the sad or guilty feelings underneath. Making sure I eat a good meal, and don't exercise in response to these feelings. Giving myself some time to feel sad.

Form 14.1
Changing Your EDBs

This worksheet is to help you generate ideas about how to engage in opposite action, rather than your customary EDBs, in response to common triggers. Articulating the possible positive consequences of the opposite action may increase your motivation to change your EDBs.

Situation/trigger	Emotion	EDB	Opposite action	Positive consequence of opposite action
Ex-husband	Sadness, guilt, worthlessness. Anger as a secondary emotion.	Diet, exercise, compl aining	Writing in journal or talking to friend about sadness	Possibly learning something new or getting a new perspective. Actually dealing with sadness instead of making myself more sad and lonely by being underweight.

Worksheet 14.3
EDB Reading and Reflection

Thinking about learned responses

Understanding what comes before our emotions are triggered (the *antecedents*, the A in ARC) helps us to better understand our emotions and our emotional *responses* (R). It is also important to understand the *consequences* (C) of our responses to emotional experiences, and in particular our emotion-driven behaviors or EDBs. We are designed to learn from our experiences. The only way for us to know what is good and what is bad is through our experiences, and our emotions help to guide us in making this distinction. If we want to ensure our survival, we should move toward things that are good for us and away from things that are bad. More often than not, it is our emotions that are telling us what is good and what is bad.

If you think about it, this serves a very adaptive purpose in nature. For example, if a rabbit in the forest comes across a fox lurking in the bushes near its favorite watering hole, the intense emotion of fear the rabbit experiences helps the rabbit to learn that it should stay away from this potentially life-threatening situation in the future. The rabbit learns very quickly from this experience of fear that in order to ensure its survival, it should probably avoid this area and would be better off finding itself a new watering hole. This type of learning takes place in nature all the time and just goes to show that even if we don't necessarily like fear, fear definitely has its place and is a very adaptive emotion.

This type of learning from uncomfortable emotions is not only for animals in the wild. It is something people share and has been passed down through evolution. As humans, we too are designed to learn quickly from our experiences. For example, if you are cooking on a stove and accidentally grab a pot handle that is very hot, you experience pain and immediately pull your hand away. When you reach for a pot handle the next time, you may stop yourself and grab a potholder instead in order to avoid the unpleasant experience of being burned again. You have learned that in order to avoid pain, you should think twice before grabbing something on the stove. What's more, we are also designed to quickly apply what we have learned not only to the immediate situation but to other similar situations as well.

You may be thinking, this is great, but what does this have to do with my symptoms? The important thing to understand here is that we have the ability to quickly learn and alter our behavior in response to unpleasant emotional experiences. For the most part, this is adaptive, but this might not always be the case. What about giving in to the EDB of escape by leaving a crowded event every time we feel panicky, even if being at the event itself is important to us? What about altering our behavior to avoid the possibility of an unpleasant experience like contracting germs on a train by refusing to take public transportation? Or how about altering our behavior to avoid the unpleasant emotion of embarrassment by avoiding all social gatherings? Sometimes we interpret our emotions as guiding us away from a threatening situation that might not even be an actual threat, and our responses in turn become maladaptive (unhelpful) instead of adaptive (helpful). Part of the aim of this program is to help you make the distinction between what is a real threat and what is a *perceived* threat, allowing you to better understand when and how emotions *should* guide you. We will discuss all of this in more detail in upcoming chapters, but for now, the important thing to begin paying attention to is how we learn from our emotional experiences.

When we experience strong emotions, they leave lasting impressions. What triggers our emotions, and what happens when we have them, stays with us and influences how we experience similar situations in the future. As humans, we also learn to repeat things that make us feel good and to avoid things that make us feel bad. However, as humans we also have the gift of reasoning and foresight; therefore, we also may learn to do certain things in order to keep ourselves from *potentially* feeling bad. For example, if spicy foods give you heartburn, you may avoid spicy foods. Similarly, if large social gatherings make you uncomfortable, you may avoid going to large social gatherings. If you don't want to wait in long lines at the supermarket, you may do your shopping late at night or during a weekday afternoon or online instead. If you are trying to write an essay and you don't want to face the possibility that you can't think of what to say, you may clean the house or watch TV rather than start to write. Similarly, if you don't want to experience a panic attack, you may walk to work instead of riding the train.

In addition to learning to avoid strong emotions, engaging in the behavior the strong emotion is driving us to do (the EDB), such as running when afraid even if there is nothing to be afraid of, forces us to learn some inappropriate, damaging responses because engaging in the EDB does serve to relieve the emotion. Thus, engaging in an EDB, even if it is for just a short time, relieves the emotion and helps us avoid feeling worse. For example, we might avoid making eye contact during conversations, or quickly exit a crowded area when feeling panicky, or stay in bed all day when feeling down. Over time, however, we learn to do this same EDB over and over again in an attempt to relieve the emotion and the possibility of feeling worse. The problem is that repeatedly doing these EDBs can result in a vicious cycle in which the EDBs become automatic, counterproductive, and inconsistent with the actual situation. Because these EDBs relieve uncomfortable emotions in the short term, we may think they are useful for us. However, they may actually be interfering in important ways with our ability to live our lives. These learned strategies for coping with intense emotions, such as avoiding situations that trigger emotions, represent the "Cs" or consequences phase of the ARC model. By avoiding these strong and intense feelings, we never have the chance to find out what these emotions might really be telling us or to see that *these emotions will pass*. Thus, by avoiding intense emotions, we may actually be depriving ourselves of important, valued aspects of our lives.

Can you think of something you have learned to do to avoid experiencing something bad? What was the experience that influenced you?

_____

_____

_____

What about something you have learned to do to experience something good? What was the experience that influenced you in this case?

_____

_____

_____

_____

Confronting Physical Sensations

GOALS

- Understand the importance of learning to tolerate physical sensations of emotion.
- Practice exercises that stimulate sensations associated with negative emotions.
- Consider other exercises that might be personally relevant to your physical sensations.
- Plan to practice those exercises daily.

HOMEWORK REVIEW

The homework from the EDB session is very important. However, we are not going to take the time at the beginning of the interoceptive exposure session to review it because we want to get started with interoceptive exposure as quickly as possible. Taking the time to review the homework may increase anticipatory anxiety about the exposure process. Instead, we will both review the homework and plan additional homework for the next session after doing the interoceptive exercises.

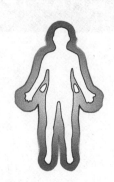

We already know that physical sensations play an important role in emotional experiences. We also have automatic thoughts associated with those sensations. For instance, when you are frightened or excited, your heart might beat more quickly. You would have different reactions to this same sensation if you interpret this harder beating as "I might be having a heart attack!" versus "I'm excited about this roller coaster!" or even "My pounding heart has been trained to occur in this type of situation." Once we have automatic *negative* interpretations of the physical sensations associated with emotion, then they can become "signs" that our emotions are more intense than they really are and can influence the intensity of our emotional response, as well as what we do in response to our emotions.

There are great examples of how our physical sensations help to trap us in negative emotional cycles. For example, it might have happened that you were nervous about eating a high-calorie food, and that you also had a stomachache at the same time. Later, you might worry that a high-calorie food would *cause* a stomachache and start to especially notice how your stomach felt—every sensation that you had would become notable, and your own anxiety might then cause the stomachache. If you know it is anxiety, as opposed to a food intolerance, it might be easier to bear. By becoming more aware of and comfortable with our internal physical sensations, we can begin to put them into perspective and see how they contribute to our emotional experience.

There are amazing examples of how physical sensations can trigger negative emotions without any conscious involvement whatsoever. For example, being anxious raises the surface temperature of our skin and makes people feel hot. If you interpret being hot as being anxious, then it is possible that just feeling hot—going into a hot room, or even having your temperature rise during sleep—can set off an anxious reaction. That is one reason why people have panic attacks in their sleep. We can't always figure out what set things off, but we can start to desensitize ourselves to the common triggers so that they are less likely to happen.

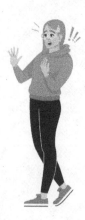

- Can you do a quick "three-point check" of your thoughts, physical sensations, and behaviors?
- Can you identify unhelpful automatic appraisals and thinking traps?
- Can you find new, more helpful ways to look at the situation?
- Are you noticing any unhelpful EDBs or avoidance strategies you are using?
- Can you replace these unhelpful EDBs and avoidance with alternative actions to lean in?

Consider your expectancies

It is also important to check your thoughts, physical sensations, and behaviors *before* doing situational exposures, and compare these with your thoughts, physical sensations, and behaviors just *after* completing the exposure.

- Were your fears and/or appraisals confirmed?
- Were your physical sensations as intense or intolerable as you had anticipated?
- Were you able to counter avoidance strategies and unhelpful EDBs?
- Ask yourself, "What did I learn from this situation?" As long as you are learning new things—the primary goal of exposure—then there is no such thing as a "failure."

What is the point of emotion exposures?

Many people—even therapists!—get confused about the point of emotion exposures. Although many people would like their emotions to be less strong, the point is *not* to reduce the experience of strong emotions—particularly not during the exposures themselves! Rather, the point of emotion exposures is *to promote tolerance of emotions through new learning, new experiences, and new behaviors over contexts and time.*

Emotion exposures will obviously vary from person to person. One of the skills we will learn in this session is how to make a list—or a hierarchy—of situations that vary in how much they provoke uncomfortable emotions. This is your chance to put your new skills into action. These skills will also help you to eliminate any emotion avoidance during these emotion exposures. Remember, engaging in emotion avoidance during these exposures will interfere with your progress during treatment. Emotion avoidance strategies not only prevent you from fully experiencing your emotions but also prevent you from learning new information about the experiences, such as your ability to cope with these experiences. In order to learn new ways of responding to emotionally intense situations, it is necessary to conduct exercises to intentionally bring on these types of emotional experiences. Emotional reactions cannot be changed until emotions are fully experienced and EDBs are identified and modified.

Creating a hierarchy: what can I expect to be doing?

In order to be in situations and activities that will help you test your skills, a lot of planning is required on your part. Your next important step is to create an *Emotional and Situational Hierarchy*, or an "exposure hierarchy." Soon you will do an exercise to get started. But before you do, it's important to understand what the goal of the hierarchy is and what goes in it.

What's the goal?

Eventually your hierarchy will be an ordered list of the types of situations that provoke uncomfortable emotions for you, and situations that you most often avoid. You will write your ordered list on Form 16.1: Fear and Avoidance Hierarchy. Take a look at the form now, along with Figure 16.2: Fear and Avoidance Hierarchy—Example (both the form and the example figure appear near the end of this chapter), and follow along during the explanation. You will "rate" the situations using a Subjective Units of Distress Scale (SUDS) from those that are moderately uncomfortable up to those that are extremely uncomfortable. When you are ready, over time, you will gradually work up from the bottom of the hierarchy to the top. You can (and should) always work on editing your hierarchy, making small changes as you experience your exposure activities.

Describe situations you are currently avoiding in order to prevent uncomfortable emotions from occurring, starting with the worst or most distressing situation. Rate the degree to which you avoid each of the situations you describe, and the degree of distress they cause.

Do Not Avoid	Hesitate to Enter Situation, But Rarely Avoid		Sometimes Avoid		Usually Avoid		Always Avoid	
0	1	2	3	4	5	6	7	8
No Distress	Slight Distress		Definite Distress		Strong Distress		Extreme Distress	

	Description	Avoid	Distress
1 WORST	Giving an emotional toast in a tight bridesmaid's dress at a wedding; large portion fettuccini alfredo, knowing I will have dessert, not having exercised that day; riding in the back seat of a cab or Uber with people next to me and someone in the front passenger seat	8	8
2	Having everyone looking at me: center of attention, public speaking; fried chicken, going back for seconds, without fasting or exercising during the day; riding in the back seat of a cab or Uber alone	8	8
3	Riding in an elevator to the top floor; riding on a busy train or bus; mashed potatoes with unknown amount of cream and butter mixed in; eating "messy" food with hands without using a napkin until the end	8	8
4	Two pieces of pizza, eating in front of other people, eating with my hands; in public; wearing tight clothes in public and eating at the same time	7	7
5	Not asking for reassurance from my parents; whole bagel with cream cheese from a large container (no measuring); leaving things undone, such as not tidying or organizing my things; wearing tight clothes in public without changing or covering up	6	6
6	Talking to people in authority; admitting my emotions; handful of pretzels from bag, dipped in hummus in a bowl	6	6
7	Looking in the mirror, shopping & trying on clothes; coffee with unknown amounts of cream and sugar pre-mixed for me	5	5
8	Maintaining conversation with someone I don't know well; ½ bagel with individual pack of cream cheese	4	4

Figure 16.2:

Fear and Avoidance Hierarchy—Example

What's in a hierarchy?

There are going to be different types of situations combined together in the hierarchy. Some areas that we recommend are body image, food, and social activities, as illustrated in Figure 16.3.

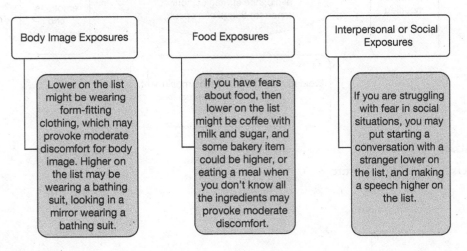

Figure 16.3:

Common Emotion Exposures

However, you may have other issues that you'll want to work on using exposure activities, such as shown in Figure 16.4.

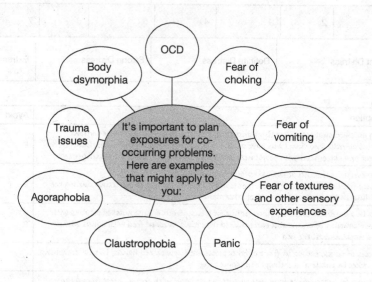

Figure 16.4:

Common Co-occurring Emotional Disorders for Emotion Exposure Hierarchy

When you fully engage in exposure, the important things shown in Figure 16.5 can happen.

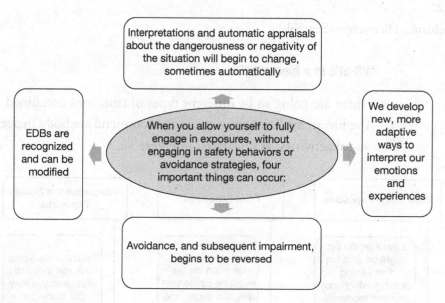

Figure 16.5:

Four Effects of Emotion Exposure

In-Session Exercise 16.1
Developing a Fear and Avoidance Hierarchy

A big factor in the success of treatment lies in your practice of emotion exposures. **You should aim to do exposure activities every day**. An important skill is being able to plan the right kind of exposure. The next step is to create your own exposure hierarchy—a list of your feared and avoided situations, consisting of various activities (situational and/or imaginal) that will elicit the uncomfortable and distressing emotions that you typically avoid. Our exercise for today is to start making that list. Just to get us started, we are going to brainstorm a list of avoided and feared situations. Don't worry too much about SUD scores and categories, or difficulty ratings. Just focus on generating a lot of different exposure ideas. Your list can be really messy because we are going to copy it over later to your Hierarchy Form. For this activity you will need Box 16.2: Hierarchy Examples Sheet and Form 16.1: Fear and Avoidance Hierarchy, both located later in this chapter.

It can be an "imaginal" exposure just to fill out the top of the hierarchy. For the things that would cause you the *most* discomfort (for example, eating a full meal of pasta without exercising afterward, singing a song in front of strangers, touching a toilet and then not washing your hands all day), just naming and writing down these things is work enough right now. Down at the bottom of the form, you should include things that you would avoid and would cause you discomfort but that you can possibly imagine actually doing. Once you have done some of the things at the bottom, it will seem more possible to do the things in the middle. Once you have done the things in the middle, it will seem more possible to do the things at the top. You do *not* have to be ready to do all these things right now!

Emotion exposures can be designed around any situation that evokes uncomfortable emotions for you, allowing you to practice emotion regulation skills you have learned (such as nonjudgmental, present-focused awareness; identifying and challenging automatic appraisals; countering emotion avoidance and EDBs; and tolerating physical sensations). When designing exposures, it is important to consider that uncomfortable emotions can be negative or positive. If there are pleasurable emotions you avoid, think how to include those in your hierarchy.

This part of treatment can be hard for people at first. But remember, you have learned *so much* from treatment that will help you tolerate and learn from emotional situations. It is in this final stage of the treatment that all that learning really pays off!

At this point, try to write down at least five things on your hierarchy sheet, dealing with different areas of your issues (food, body image, other issues). If you have lots of ideas, go ahead and write them all down. Try to come up with ones that would be more and less difficult to actually do—from things you can imagine doing that would be a little challenging, all the way up to things that it is almost impossible to imagine doing.

Here is a list of some principles to refer to when conducting emotion exposures:

1. **Provoke the "right" amount of emotion.**
   - Start with exposures that are low to moderate intensity, and progress higher as you go.
   - Don't be afraid to modify exposures in the moment.
   - Use interoceptive exercises before exposure to increase the emotional intensity.

2. **Stay with the emotion (mindfulness).**
   - Lean into the emotion; try to experience it fully.
   - Report SUDS scores periodically throughout.
   - Anticipate, identify, and remove avoidance and safety signals as they arise.

3. **Set reasonable goals and review new learning after the exposure.**
   - Report expectancies—identify thinking traps.
   - Review whether expectancies were confirmed.
   - Identify successes! Reappraise "failures."
   - Congratulate yourself for even trying to do something so difficult!

Why are expectancies so important?

Expectancies are what we expect, which means they are the automatic appraisals we have in anticipation of something. Anticipatory anxiety is very powerful. When we think about going into a challenging situation, we have anticipatory anxiety, and this anxiety shapes the thoughts we have about what it is going to be like.

Let's think of the example of riding in an elevator. Someone who is getting ready to go into the elevator might have expectancies such as *I'm going to be terrified, I am going to feel sick to my stomach and possibly vomit, I might faint, This elevator could get stuck and what if I can't get help?* and so on. These thoughts are important to identify, and it is also important to briefly examine these appraisals using the skills you have: Are these overly catastrophic? Are you overestimating the probability that these will happen? If it actually happened, could you cope?

What about the example of going to a busy café and sitting alone while having a coffee and a pastry? What might your expectancies be if this were you? Are these overly catastrophic? Are they overestimating the probability that these will happen? If it actually happened, could you cope?

Then, when the exposure is over, you should re-examine your expectancies and see whether they came true, and if you were able to cope. There is a form called Form 16.2: Record of Emotion Exposure, shown later in this chapter, which we will review very briefly together now. There is also an example of the form already filled out (Box 16.1: Record of Emotion Exposure Practice—Mock Example) to use for reference. Form 16.2 is what you will use before and after every planned exposure activity.

Looking out for avoidance and safety signals

Hopefully you have come to be aware of your own methods of cognitive and behavioral avoidance over the course of the program so far and have developed nonjudgmental awareness skills. For an exposure to be successful, it is important to try *not* to avoid the emotional experience. In fact, the more intense you can allow the experience to be, the better! We have a saying that in exposures, we look for the discomfort and the fear, and then we go after it. If you avoid, you come out the other side thinking things like:

- *I made it, but the only reason was because I sang "Dixie" to myself the whole time.*
- *I made it, but only because the picture of my mom in my pocket kept me feeling safe.*
- *I made it, but it was pure luck this time; it wouldn't happen that way for me again.*

The thought that you would never have made it through "*if it hadn't been for this or that*" is just the opposite of what we want to learn! We want to learn that we can have intense emotional experiences and they will be OK, they will pass, and we can deal with them without trying to make those feelings less intense, or protecting ourselves from them by using avoidance strategies in our usual ways. Therefore, if you realize that you are using avoidance during an exposure, you should try to remove that behavior or avoidance strategy as quickly as possible.

Staying in the situation long enough

If you remember the graph of how emotion rises and falls (Figure 10.1), way back when we were learning about emotion, we develop patterns of avoidance by escaping the situation before the emotion starts to pass naturally. One goal of emotion exposure planning is to arrange situations where you can stay in the situation long enough 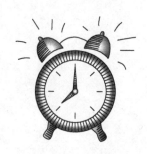 for the emotion to really get to a peak and then start to come down, ideally by about 50%, or down to a SUDS rating of around 3. These are just guidelines, and it is possible to have a very successful exposure, and learn a lot, without this taking place. But what you do *not* want to do is plan something that intentionally or unintentionally involves escaping quickly, before you have had time to bring on the emotion, tolerate it, and learn something from it.

Why is repetition important?

One of the most important principles to keep in mind is that emotion exposures need to be repeated. Learning new lessons about emotion takes time and practice—the old lessons were learned over many repetitions, and the new lessons need repetition as well. Emotion exposures become 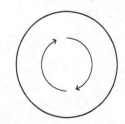 easier over multiple repetitions: You know what to expect, you adjust to the situation, and you learn you can cope. An exposure can be adjusted for the next repetition. If it was not stimulating enough, you can up the challenge a bit, or if it was very hard, you can think about how to create supports that will allow you to immerse yourself more completely.

Therapists doing exposure therapy for anxiety disorders often show their clients a graph, like the one in Figure 16.6, of how anxiety may decrease over time with repeated exposures. In actual therapy, your emotions will probably not change in exactly this way. But you can expect that some things will change and improve with repeated exposure if you try to apply the principles that are described here.

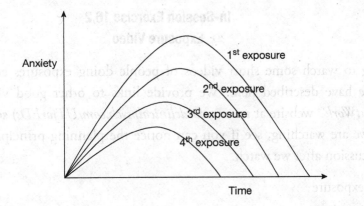

Figure 16.6:

Classic Graph of Repeated Exposures for Anxiety

In-Session Exercise 16.2
Exposure Video

We are going to watch some short videos of people doing exposures according to the principles that we have described here. We provide links to other good videos as well (on the *TreatmentsThatWork*™ website at *www.oxfordclinicalpsych.com/UTforEDs*) so you can watch them later. While we are watching, see if you can notice the planning principles that we've covered today, for discussion after we watch.

- Coffee exposure
- Flying exposure
- Messy finger-food exposure
- Elevator exposure
- Social exposure

Before we leave the session, you should commit to doing one exposure on your hierarchy.

Explanation of this session's homework

In the remaining weeks of this treatment, you will focus on conducting exposures both in session and out of session. Session time will be devoted to planning and conducting emotion exposures as well as reviewing exposures that you have done out of session.

Homework

Many of the forms and worksheets will need to be filled out more than once. We are including one blank copy of every worksheet and form for you. For those items that you will need more than once, your therapist will provide additional copies, or you can download blank copies yourself from the TreatmentsThatWork™ website at www.oxfordclinicalpsych.com/ UTforEDs.

- Fill out Form 3.1: Eating, Depression, and Anxiety (EDA).
- Plot scores on Form 3.2: EDA Graph.
- Fill out Form 4.1: Regular Eating Food Log.
- Complete Form 8.1: The ARC of Emotional Experiences.
- **One emotion exposure:** _____
    - Complete Form 16.2: Record of Emotion Exposure.
    - Repeat same exposure at least twice!
- Continue filling in Form 16.1: Fear and Avoidance Hierarchy; if needed, review Figure 16.2: Fear and Avoidance Hierarchy—Example and Box 16.2: Hierarchy Examples Sheet.
- Watch videos of emotion exposures.

Form 16.1
Fear and Avoidance Hierarchy

Describe situations you are currently avoiding in order to prevent uncomfortable emotions from occurring, starting with the worst or most distressing situation. Rate the degree to which you avoid each of the situations you describe, and the degree of distress they cause.

Do Not Avoid	Hesitate to Enter But Rarely Avoid			Sometimes Avoid		Usually Avoid		Always Avoid
0	1	2	3	4	5	6	7	8
No Distress		Slight Distress		Definite Distress		Strong Distress		Extreme Distress
	Description						Avoid	Distress
1 WORST								
2								
3								
4								
5								
6								
7								
8								
9								
10								
11								
12								
13								
14								
15								

Box 16.1
Record of Emotion Exposure Practice—Mock Example

Exposure Task: <u>wearing tight clothes in public without changing or covering up</u>

Prior to the task:

Anticipatory Distress (0–8): <u>6</u>

Thoughts, Feelings, and Behaviors you noticed before the task:

<u>My tummy fat will be bulging out, everyone will be staring at me, I will feel very self-conscious and embarrassed about how I look, I will fold my arms or hide my tummy with my bag, I will feel tearful and will be blushing; I will be sweating so much that my armpit sweat will be soaking and noticeable through my t-shirt.</u>

Re-evaluate your automatic appraisals about the task:

<u>I doubt anyone will be staring at me; in fact some people won't even notice me; my tummy and skin will not bulge because even though the clothes are form-fitting, they are actually the right size for my body; if I notice an urge to use avoidance behaviors I'll talk about it first; if I feel tearful, or blush, or if I feel embarrassed I will lean in to these experiences and allow them to rise and peak and fall; I might sweat due to feeling anxious, but my t-shirt will likely not become "soaked."</u>

<u>After completing the task:</u>

Thoughts, Feelings, and Behaviors you noticed during the task:

<u>That was not as bad as I thought; nobody noticed me and nobody stared; the clothes were not as uncomfortable as I thought; I did not get tearful at all; I did feel embarrassed and blushed at the beginning, but those sensations subsided quickly; I resisted folding my arms; I think I did sweat, but I didn't notice it much.</u>

Number of minutes you did the task: <u>1 hour</u>

Maximum distress during the task (0–8): <u>6</u>

Distress at the end of the task (0–8): <u>3 or even 2</u>

Any attempts to avoid your emotions (distraction, safety signals, etc.)?

<u>Lots of urges to use avoidance strategies! I reminded myself to not use avoidance as each urge came up. I did notice myself avoiding eye contact when I spoke to</u>

someone in the mall, and my anxiety spiked quickly and then fell again after a few moments.

What did you take away from this exposure task? Did your feared outcomes occur? If so, how were you able to cope with them?

My expectancies were disproven; I tolerated my distress; I leaned in without using my safety signals. Next time I'll work on eye contact and stay in the situation for longer.

Form 16.2
Record of Emotion Exposure

Exposure Task:

_____

Prior to the task:

Anticipatory Distress (0–8): _____

Thoughts, Feelings, and Behaviors you noticed before the task:

_____

_____

Re-evaluate your automatic appraisals about the task:

_____

_____

After completing the task:

Thoughts, Feelings, and Behaviors you noticed during the task:

_____

_____

Number of minutes you did the task: _____

Maximum distress during the task (0–8): _____

Distress at the end of the task (0–8): _____

Any attempts to avoid your emotions (distraction, safety signals, etc.)?

_____

_____

What did you learn? Did your feared outcomes occur? Were you able to cope?

_____

_____

Box 16.2
Hierarchy Examples Sheet

Every individual's list of uncomfortable situations is personal and different. It may be helpful to think of the following areas when creating your personal hierarchy. Make them personal, though; include the particular things that are specific that you avoid or would make you uncomfortable.

Food and eating

Eating foods with unknown ingredients
Eating foods of known high fat content/known high calories
Eating particular feared foods
Eating more than other people

Examples

- *Choose a pasta dish for lunch*
- *Eat pizza for dinner*
- *Have chips or fries with sandwich*
- *Put an oil-based condiment on sandwich (mayo, ranch dressing)*
- *Have chocolate milk at lunch*
- *Choose an oil-based dressing for salad*
- *Choose a hamburger over a turkey burger*
- *Add a 4th dessert for the week*
- *Have juice with a meal*
- *Pick a sesame bagel instead of a wheat bagel*
- *Put chickpeas, corn, or avocado in salad*
- *Add a banana at dinner*
- *Cook a dish with butter and sugar*

Body image and body dysmorphic disorder

Looking at your body in a mirror
Displaying your body (not hiding it)
Allowing your body (or body parts) to be seen in "unflattering" situations
Displaying or highlighting the "flawed" body part

Examples

- *Go swimming in the school pool*
- *Shop for bathing suits at the mall*
- *Take a picture and post it on social media unfiltered, unmanipulated*

214

- *Take an unattractive picture of yourself and don't delete it*
- *Wear exercise clothes that show your stomach at the gym*
- *Wear jeans and close-fitting top to school*
- *Look in the mirror while wearing shorts*
- *Look in less-flattering mirror*
- *See your weight on a scale*
- *Imagine your weight on a scale in great detail*
- *Go outside without makeup or with messy hair*
- *Wear a t-shirt with no sleeves while walking the dog*

Social anxiety

Talking to stranger
Public speaking
Not following the rules for "getting along" (e.g., disagreeing, asking for favors)
Talking to authority figures
Doing something embarrassing

Examples

- *Give a presentation in front of strangers on a topic you aren't prepared for (videotape it)*
- *Sing a song outside a store*
- *Ask a stranger for directions to a place that doesn't exist*
- *Ask a stranger to take a photograph of you*
- *Speak to an attractive person at the mall*
- *Ask the store clerk to get you several items in different sizes*
- *Ask an authority figure (teacher, policeman) for a favor*
- *Send the food back at a restaurant*
- *Eat a meal in public*
- *Go to a party and stay for 1 hour*
- *Make a phone call in front of someone else*
- *Come in late to class and walk in front of other students*
- *Sit in the middle or front of class*
- *Make small talk with people in line at a coffee shop*
- *Role play doing a job interview*
- *Say something in class*

Obsessive-compulsive disorder/perfectionism

Violating symmetry and order rules (making things disorganized, messy)
Touching dirty things without washing hands

Deliberately failing at something, leaving something unfinished, making mistakes
Watching television or reading books on topics that are related to intrusive thoughts

Examples of contamination exposures (within reason and CDC guidelines)

- *Touch a toilet and don't wash hands*
- *Touch a subway wall and don't wash hands*
- *Drink from someone else's glass or water bottle*
- *Eat food from a buffet*
- *Walk on public floor with bare feet*
- *Ride on the subway and touch things after other people do*
- *Use a public toilet*
- *Eat nonorganic food*
- *Go out without hand sanitizer*
- *Shake hands with a stranger*

Examples of perfectionism exposures

- *Post a message on social media with a typo in it*
- *Post a message on social media that admits to a mistake*
- *Send an email with a typo in it*
- *Submit a paper with two pages out of order*
- *Leave the house a mess when a friend comes over*
- *Ask for an extension on an assignment or tell someone you couldn't do something on time*
- *Go outside with clothing and hair in disarray*

Panic/agoraphobia/claustrophobia/depersonalization

Being in a crowd, physically touching other people
Being in a small, enclosed space
Being in a wide-open, brightly lit space
Drinking caffeinated beverages or being hot

Examples of panic exposures

- *Sit in a movie theatre in a middle seat, away from exits*
- *Ride on crowded public transportation*
- *Go somewhere underground (subway, small basement room) and closed in*
- *Watch a scary movie without looking away*
- *Drink caffeine, exercise, and sit in a crowded space*

Specific phobias (we include just two specific examples here)

Spending extended time in direct contact with phobic object
Spending time with phobic object physically separated (in a box, across the room)
Interacting with fake version of phobic object (plastic, toy, simulated)
Watching media (cartoon, shows, movies) about phobic object
Looking at line drawings or cartoons of phobic object
Thinking about phobic object or looking at the word on a page
Saying the name of the phobic object

Examples of vomiting phobia exposures

- *Mix together condiments and milk and put it in the toilet*
- *Simulate retching*
- *Visit someone who is sick*
- *Sit in a pediatrician's waiting room, touch the walls, use the bathroom (don't wash hands)*
- *Watch YouTube videos of people vomiting*
- *Go on rides at an amusement park*
- *Role play vomiting with sounds of vomiting*
- *Go on a trip to a foreign place*
- *Eat at an unfamiliar restaurant*
- *Look at a cartoon of a character vomiting*
- *Look at the word "vomit" on a piece of paper*
- *Put food in your mouth and spit it into the toilet*
- *Drink a glass of wine*

Examples of spider phobia exposures

- *Let a tarantula crawl on your arm*
- *Hold a box with a spider in it*
- *From across the room, look at a box with a spider in it*
- *Go to the zoo and look at spiders*
- *Go to a natural history museum and look at taxidermied spiders*
- *Watch media (movies, TV shows) about spiders*
- *Have a plastic spider on your arm, on your face*
- *Look at a very detailed photograph of a spider*
- *Think about a spider*
- *Say the word "spider"*

Relapse Prevention

GOALS

- Review the important takeaway messages of this program.
- Evaluate your progress.
- Revisit your treatment goals.
- Develop a practice plan.

HOMEWORK REVIEW

- Fill out Form 3.1: Eating, Depression, and Anxiety (EDA).
- Plot scores on Form 3.2: EDA Graph.
- Fill out Form 4.1: Regular Eating Food Log.
- Complete Form 8.1: The ARC of Emotional Experiences.
- One emotion exposure: _____
  - Complete Form 16.2: Record of Emotion Exposure
  - Repeat same exposure at least twice!
- Continue filling in Form 16.1: Fear and Avoidance Hierarchy; if needed, review Figure 16.2: Fear and Avoidance Hierarchy–Example and Box 16.2: Hierarchy Examples Sheet.
- Watch videos of emotion exposures.

The main point of this session is to review key concepts from this treatment program and to prepare you for what comes next.[1] We will review strategies that will help you continue to strengthen the skills you have been practicing.

Here are the important takeaways from this program for you to remember:

- All emotions, even the ones that feel negative or uncomfortable, are providing you with information that can motivate you to take action in helpful ways.
- Staying present in the moment and taking a nonjudgmental view of your emotions can help to prevent emotions from increasing in intensity.
- The way you think about a situation influences how you feel, and how you feel affects the way you interpret a situation.
- Although avoiding uncomfortable emotion experiences can work well in the short term, it isn't an effective long-term coping strategy.

To help you remember all the skills contained in this program, we have summarized them in Box 17.1: Emotion Skills Action Plan, which you can use whenever you notice an emotion starting to build. The Emotion Skills Action Plan is rooted in the three components of an emotion to help you remember it. To keep your Emotion Skills Action Plan handy, you can make a photocopy of these steps or download a copy from the *Treatments That Work*™ website at *www.oxfordclinicalpsych.com/UTforEDs*. Alternatively, some people take a picture of the Emotion Skills Action Plan with their cellphone so that it is easily accessible anytime they are experiencing confusing emotions or the desire to engage in emotion-driven behaviors.

---

[1] The material in this chapter is largely reprinted from the UP manual, Barlow et al., 2018.

Do a quick 3-point check. Use your breath or other chosen cue as an anchor to help bring you out of your head and to anchor yourself in the present moment.

What are you thinking right now? What negative automatic thoughts are you having right now? Are you jumping to conclusions or thinking the worst? Are you responding to a past concern or future worry? Ask yourself whether there are any other ways to interpret this situation that may be more helpful and what are some ways you can cope.

What are you feeling in your body right now? What physical sensations are you noticing? Are you tired, hungry, or rundown? Are your physical sensations intensifying your emotions, or vice versa? Try to stay in the present moment with your physical sensations without trying to control them or to distract yourself.

What are you doing now, or what do you feel like doing right now? Are you avoiding a situation that may trigger an uncomfortable emotion? Remember that countering an emotional behavior involves provoking emotions and engaging in helpful Alternative Actions.

Evaluating your progress

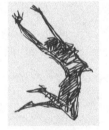

As you approach the end of this treatment program, you may be feeling excited because you've seen improvements in your symptoms. You may also be feeling disappointed that you haven't seen as much improvement or the type of changes that you had hoped. It is important to remember that the goal of completing this treatment program is to teach you skills for responding to your emotions in a more helpful way. Although it is very common for people to feel that they have made some noticeable progress in addressing their symptoms, there is often still room for improvement following this short-term treatment. This is because it takes time after learning the skills to see the full effect. Studies on this treatment have shown that clients continue to see additional improvements in their symptoms for up to a full year after completing it. It is helpful to keep this in mind as you reflect on how your symptoms have changed, and as you think about your plans to keep up the good work in the future.

There are several ways that you can evaluate the progress you've made since you began this program. One option is to take a look at Form 3.2: EDA

Graph. If you have completed the EDA and charted it on the graph, you can look at the changes over time.

You can also use Worksheet 17.1: Progress Evaluation, located later in this chapter, to reflect on the progress you have made toward learning new ways of coping with intense, uncomfortable emotions. It is important to set aside time to complete this evaluation thoughtfully. By generating specific examples of how each skill has been helpful, you will be reinforcing the connection in your brain between using the skills and positive changes in your life. We will also ask you to consider where there are opportunities for continued improvement for each skill, which will be helpful in creating Worksheet 17.2: Practice Plan, located later in this chapter.

How to maintain your progress and your momentum

As you approach the end of this treatment program, you may find yourself looking forward to taking a break. After all, treatment is hard work! However, consider Newton's first law of motion—an object at rest stays at rest and an object in motion stays in motion. Right now you are an object in motion! In other words, it is much easier to maintain all of the positive momentum that you've worked so hard to accumulate over these past months than it is to get back on track after taking a break. Next we recommend strategies for maintaining your progress and continuing to benefit from treatment.

Revisit your goals

In Chapter 4, you came up with some goals for treatment. Setting goals is a critical part of making changes to your life and maintaining your motivation. Take a look back at Worksheet 4.1: "Taking the Necessary Steps" Homework Sheet, which you completed at the start of this program. Now that you have completed this  treatment, you may have made significant progress on some of the goals you set. In order to stay motivated, it can be helpful to take a minute to revisit your goals and update them if necessary. Now that you're feeling better, more possibilities may seem open to you—like starting to date, going back to school, or getting a new job.

When updating your goals, remember that people tend to feel most motivated when working toward something that is important to them. So choose those goals that are personally meaningful to you. Once you have updated goals in mind, ask yourself the following:

- Are my goals specific and concrete enough for me to easily measure my progress?
- Are my goals manageable and realistic? The purpose of goals is to motivate you, and if you set goals that are unrealistic, you could end up feeling defeated.
- Is the ability to achieve my goals within my control, or is the outcome dependent on reasons beyond my control? For example, if you set a goal to go on two job interviews next month, there are many reasons outside your control why that may not be achievable. However, if your goal is to submit two job applications, it is much more under your control!

Create a practice plan

The single most effective way to maintain the progress you have made in this program and to keep improving is to continue to practice the skills you have learned. Keep in mind that even if you have made significant progress so far, these are newly learned behaviors that will require time and effort in order to "stick."

Worksheet 17.2: Practice Plan is designed to help you come up with specific strategies for practicing each of the core skills. Studies have shown that people are more likely to take action when they plan it out in advance. First, the practice plan asks you to think about how each of the treatment skills relates to your long-term treatment goals. For example, if your long-term goal is to improve your relationships with your friends, practicing cognitive flexibility may stop you from jumping to conclusions when a friend doesn't respond to a text message.

The practice plan also asks you to come up with a plan for how you can practice each skill. Even with the best of intentions, it is hard to follow through with a practice plan unless you get specific about exactly how and when you will practice. For example, someone may plan to work on countering emotional avoidance by not using distraction as a coping strategy during the commute to work. However, that practice plan doesn't specify when or how this person will stop using distraction. Here is a better practice plan: "When I take the subway to and from work, I won't listen to music or read on my phone to distract myself. At each subway stop, I will take a deep breath to anchor myself in the present moment and do a three-point check."

Lastly, the practice plan asks you to come up with a way of holding yourself accountable for following through on your plan. There are many ways that you can hold yourself accountable. You can enlist the help of a friend or family member—sometimes just knowing that someone is going to ask you whether you followed through with your practice plan can motivate you to do it. You can also link your practice plan to other daily behaviors. For example, you could say that you aren't going to brush your teeth in the morning until you complete your straw-breathing exercises. You can also consider whether there are any steps you can take to make it easier to stick with your practice plan. For example, for the person who is planning not to listen to music or read on the phone, it may be helpful to leave headphones at home and to keep the phone powered off for the commute. A completed example of the practice plan can be seen in Table 17.1, located near the end of this chapter. If you would like additional space to develop your practice plan, you can make photocopies of Worksheet 17.2 or download it from the *Treatments That Work*™ website at *www.oxfordclinicalpsych.com/UTforEDs*.

Be your own coach

It is important that you take ownership over your continued progress. Many people find it helpful to schedule time to review their progress and revise their practice plan on a weekly basis. We recommend blocking out this time on your calendar, the same way you would for a doctor's appointment or a work meeting.

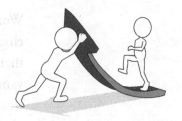

It is often said that the best offense is a strong defense, and the same is true when it comes to monitoring your symptoms. Many people wait until their symptoms start to disrupt their lives again before they make time to address them. However, if you establish the routine of checking in with yourself each week, you will be able to notice any changes in your symptoms before they get out of hand. For example, if you notice that you are starting to avoid situations that trigger intense emotions, you can proactively address this using your practice plan.

It can also be helpful to consider whether there are any upcoming situations that may be particularly challenging for you. You can anticipate some of the negative automatic thoughts that are likely to arise and the urges that you have to engage in emotion-driven behaviors. For example, big social events like weddings and reunions often cause people with a history of eating disorders to want to restrict and to notice negative automatic thoughts about what people will think about them. There are certain times of the year—like final examinations, or the end of the budgetary year, or the holidays—that bring up certain feelings. You can try to generate more flexible interpretations for your automatic thoughts and create preemptive plans for alternative actions for your urges to engage in emotion-driven behaviors ahead of time. When your emotions are likely to be especially intense, planning your coping strategy in advance can make it easier to actually use it in the moment.

Anticipating difficulties and managing setbacks

Regardless of the gains you have made in treatment, it is very likely that you will experience intense or uncomfortable emotions at times in the future! Emotional ups and downs are part of everyday life. You may notice that when you are under stress, your symptoms tend to flare up. This is very normal and similar to the way stress can affect your immune system. Sometimes, however, it may seem like your symptoms flare up when there hasn't been any increase in stress, which can be distressing. These fluctuations in symptoms are natural and normal—they do not necessarily mean you have relapsed.

The skills that you have learned to manage your emotions in more helpful ways are also applicable to coping with the inevitable ups and downs that will happen over time. For example, responding to an increase in symptoms with criticism and judgment will only intensify the symptoms. It is very easy to start jumping to conclusions and thinking the worst when symptoms flare up. You may find yourself thinking that treatment failed or you will never be able to cope with intense emotions. Your mindful emotion awareness and cognitive flexibility skills can be very helpful at these moments.

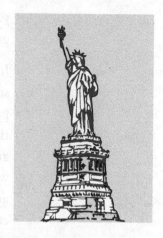

It takes time and effort to change the way you respond to your emotions, and it is hard work. Try to remember that you didn't develop these unhelpful ways of coping with intense emotions overnight, and it is unrealistic to expect they will be completely eliminated in a few months. However, with consistent practice, you will be able to replace unhelpful coping strategies with more useful ones, and change the way you respond to your emotions. The end of treatment is just the beginning of making more substantial changes in your life. To quote Michelangelo, "Every block of stone has a statue inside it and it is the task of the sculptor to discover it." You are the sculptor and you now have the tools—it's your chance now to carve the stone.

Worksheet 17.1
Progress Evaluation

Mindful emotion awareness

What are some specific improvements you've noticed in your ability to stay present in the moment instead of getting caught up in the past or worrying about the future? What are some specific improvements you've noticed in your ability to nonjudgmentally observe your emotions and your reactions to them? In what ways have you found this skill helpful?

_____

_____

_____

_____

Where do you see room for continued improvement? Are there situations where you find it more difficult to stay in the present moment or not to judge your emotional experiences? What can you do to address these challenges?

_____

_____

_____

_____

_____

Cognitive flexibility

What are some specific improvements you've noticed in your ability to be more flexible in the way you think about situations? Are you jumping to conclusions or blowing things out of proportion less often? How has this skill been useful?

_____

_____

_____

Where do you see room for continued improvement? Are there situations where you find it more difficult to be flexible in your thinking and stay out of thinking traps? What can you do to address these challenges?

_____

_____

_____

_____

Confronting physical sensations

What are some specific improvements you've noticed in your ability to respond to the physical sensations that are associated with your intense emotions? Are you doing activities that you previously avoided due to uncomfortable physical sensations? How has this skill been useful?

_____

_____

_____

_____

Where do you see room for continued improvement? Are there certain physical sensations that you still find highly distressing? What can you do to address these challenges?

_____

_____

_____

_____

Countering emotional avoidance

What are some specific improvements you've noticed in your ability to identify your unhelpful—avoidance or emotion-driven—behaviors and replace them with alternative actions? How has this skill been useful?

_____

_____

_____

_____

_____

Where do you see room for continued improvement? Are there situations where you find it more difficult replace avoidance and emotion-driven behavior with alternative actions? What can you do to address these challenges?

Table 17.1

Example Practice Plan

Use this form to generate a plan for continuing to practice these these skills after you have completed this program.

	Mindful Emotion Awareness	Cognitive Flexibility	Confronting Physical Sensations	Countering Avoidance and Emotion-Driven Behaviors
How will practicing this skill help you achieve your long-term goals?	If I remain mindful and nonjudgmental about emotion, I can notice earlier when I am feeling insecure about my body and avoid relapse.	If I can talk myself through my judgments about myself and jumping to conclusions about what others think, I will feel better about my appearance. Also I will be more willing to be social.	If I tolerate and work through the stomachaches and nausea that I have, it will be easier to eat and also easier to tolerate uncomfortable social situations.	I need to stay in social situations where I am uncomfortable and I need to continue to eat regularly even when I feel like I have eaten too much, so that I can keep getting over my social anxiety and eating disorder.
What is your specific practice plan for this skill?	If I have a strong reaction to my appearance I am going to stop and take a minute to breathe and think.	I am going to question my judgments about myself and my jumping to conclusions about what others think. Also I am going to tell my friend Sara what my jumping to conclusions are.	I'm going to keep spinning, drinking a lot of water, and not escaping from situations where I have a stomachache. I'm going to remind myself that it is from anxiety.	My new job includes conference calls and meetings, which I am not going to avoid, and I'll lean in. I'm going to keep up my regular eating plan and try to make two social plans outside of work each week. Also I'm going to try dating.
How can you hold yourself accountable to your practice plan?	When I see my therapist for a follow-up session I will check in about it. I'm also going to write in my journal about it.	I'm going to tell Sara now that I am going to tell her—also I am going to keep track of my thoughts in a journal.	I am going to tell my therapist to check in about it and I'm also going to join a Zumba class even though it aggravates my stomach.	I am going to let my boss know I have anxiety about the calls and meetings and that I am making it a work goal to speak in every meeting.

Worksheet 17.2
Practice Plan

Use this form to generate a plan for continuing to practice these skills after you have completed this program.

	Mindful Emotion Awareness	Cognitive Flexibility	Confronting Physical Sensations	Countering Avoidance and Emotion–Driven Behaviors
How will practicing this skill help you achieve your long-term goals?				
What is your specific practice plan for this skill?				
How can you hold yourself accountable to your practice plan?